Bev Aisbett is the author and illustrator of several highly regarded self-help texts for sufferers of anxiety and depression, most notably *Living with IT* and *Taming the Black Dog*. These books are distributed to health professionals nationwide and have been translated into four languages.

A trained counsellor, Bev is also the facilitator of the Art of Anxiety recovery program in Melbourne. For those unable to attend her workshop in person, she offers a home study version, *The Art of Anxiety DVD Workshop*, as well as other online resources and services. She conducts lectures to assist sufferers of depression and anxiety within metropolitan and regional Victoria.

Bev is also a recognised artist and her soulful paintings have been regularly exhibited in Victoria and Tasmania.

Workshop and lecture information,
and other anxiety resources:
www.bevaisbettartofanxiety.com

BY BEV AISBETT

Living IT Up

Letting IT Go

Get Real

Taming the Black Dog

The Little Book of IT

Fixing IT

Recovery: A Journey to Healing

The Book of IT

Get Over IT

I Love Me

All of IT: A Memoir

Living with IT

30 Days 30 Ways to Overcome Anxiety

30 DAYS 30 WAYS

TO OVERCOME ANXIETY

HarperCollins*Publishers*

HarperCollins*Publishers*

First published in Australia in 2018
by HarperCollins*Publishers* Australia Pty Limited
ABN 36 009 913 517
harpercollins.com.au

HarperCollins*Publishers*
Level 13, 201 Elizabeth Street, Sydney NSW 2000, Australia
Unit D1, 63 Apollo Drive, Rosedale, Auckland 0632, New Zealand
A 53, Sector 57, Noida, UP, India
1 London Bridge Street, London, SE1 9GF, United Kingdom
Bay Adelaide Centre, East Tower, 22 Adelaide Street West, 41st floor, Toronto,
    Ontario M5H 4E3, Canada
195 Broadway, New York NY 10007, USA

ISBN: 978 1 4607 5787 1 (pbk)

Front cover and internal illustrations by Bev Aisbett
Cover design by Hazel Lam, HarperCollins Design Studio
Typeset in Brandon Grotesque by Kelli Lonergan

DEDICATION

To my dear friends,
teachers and helpers,
without whom
I would be a reader of this
instead of the writer.

INTRODUCTION

It's taken me 25 years of practice to show you how to overcome anxiety in 30 days, so you have the *easy* part!

Contained in this book is the best of all that has been tried and tested over those 25 years — firstly, through my own journey out of severe anxiety; and, secondly, through steering all my wonderful workshop participants and one-to-one clients on the same path — to freedom from anxiety — by learning how to be their own counsellor and build their own recovery.

You might think 30 days isn't much time to overcome what may have been years of struggle, but it's not all that different from giving up any habit that isn't good for you. Once you see it in perspective, it only takes one decision to let it go.

Essentially, all that's happened is that you've had a problem but not the resources to deal with it effectively.

Overcoming anxiety isn't about *wishful* thinking — it's about employing *skilful* thinking. Without those skills, your mind can take you wherever it likes and, with anxiety, it can take you to the wildest and (let's be honest) most ridiculous places!

Now it's time for you to take back the reins and gain mastery over your own wellbeing.

Working your way through the 30 days will help you build the skills to do this one step at a time; and, like building a house, you do it in stages.

Keep your eyes on the prize and stick with it. If you conk out after Day 10, you're only going to have the slab and a couple of walls done!

Look at it this way. You head off on a road trip because you want to get to the destination. Do you get halfway then turn around and go home because you're frustrated that you haven't arrived yet?

And consider this — maybe you haven't arrived yet because you keep taking detours into things that bog you down!

You could approach the 30 days and make it hard work, or you could approach it with interest and enthusiasm. But whichever way you do it, just do it, eh? You are going to be living out the next 30 days anyway, so you may as well do something useful with them.

Making these skills super-effective means using them until they become second nature. You're getting a taste of how much better you can feel by trying them for 30 days. To make them really stick, ideally you'll make them a part of your ongoing normal routine.

Having said that, any one of these 30-day practices could have you turning the corner because each day's focus contains an insight into yourself.

It's not your anxiety that has to change: it's how you use your anxiety to help you change that leads to healing.

You might do your 30 days on a daily basis; or you might reserve one day a week, when you don't have other distractions, to give the practices your full attention.

It's up to you. There's no 'have to' about this. But if you choose to undertake the journey over 30 days, you can feel sooo much better in just a month's time!

Oh, and by the way — if you are not familiar with 'IT' from my previous books, here he is ...

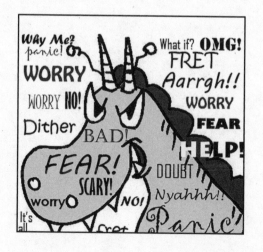

I created 'IT' to represent that worrisome, critical inner voice that generates anxiety.

He's actually not a bad guy; he's just a little *overly-vigilant* — but, yes, his presence and messages can seem scary at first till you better understand what's really going on and how to work with him.

Over the 30 days, you'll come to see him in a different and much kinder light.

My love and best wishes to you,
Bev XXX

DAY 1

You are not BROKEN

You are not being PUNISHED

Good, Kind,
Successful & Attractive People
can get ANXIETY too!

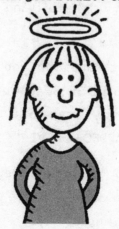

Your EMOTIONAL BAROMETER needs adjustment. Your THINKING THERMOMETER is overheated.

Think of a car. If you run it on watered-down petrol, fail to maintain it properly, let it overheat and run it into the ground, would you be surprised if it stopped working properly or started to give you 'trouble'?

Well, that's all that's happening to you!

If you have spent a lifetime (consciously or unconsciously) feeding yourself thoughts of DOOM and GLOOM, if you CRITICISED and JUDGED yourself harshly, and/or if you expected the WORST and LAMENTED the past, you were creating a 'PERFECT STORM' which translates to ANXIETY. You couldn't help it — it's just the way you did things; nonetheless, that's why you're ANXIOUS.

Mystery solved! It's just STRESS! And you don't handle stress WELL, do you?

So please let go of the idea that you have some HORRIBLE, INCURABLE DISEASE that has appeared out of NOWHERE, or that you can do NOTHING about this, or that you are TRAPPED FOREVER!

You now need to MANAGE your anxiety. And that's what we're about to start doing. Are you BEATING YOURSELF UP for having anxiety?

Are you telling yourself you're WEAK or STUPID, or that you've LOST EVERYTHING because you feel this way?

Why are you TURNING on yourself? Is that going to help you feel LESS ANXIOUS? NO! So CUT that OUT!

For Pete's sake, how could you do it any other way if you hadn't yet LEARNED how to? Would you expect a person with no carpentry skills to build you a perfect piece of furniture? NO!

Actually, if you've experienced any SHOCKS, LOSSES or TRAUMA in your past (especially in childhood) or if you are HIGHLY SENSITIVE (most anxious people are!), it would be more surprising if you DIDN'T feel anxious!

Most of us fumble our way through life by TRIAL and ERROR, without any real road map on how to manage our emotional wellbeing.

Few of us are taught *emotional intelligence*. We learn from those who have influence in our lives but who are not necessarily IDEAL mentors!

All that's happening is that you now have evidence that whatever you've been doing hasn't been WORKING FOR YOU, so it's time to gain some more EFFECTIVE skills!

Learning any new skill can feel ODD or AWKWARD at first. You're sure you'll NEVER get the hang of it! But eventually you do, don't you? Especially if you REALLY want it.

'Of course I want it!' I hear you protest. 'Why would I want to stay feeling like this?'

Well, people get used to FEELING BAD. Feeling bad becomes a HABIT and it can feel strangely COMFORTABLE, simply because it's FAMILIAR. When breaking any HABIT, you need to be COMMITTED to moving on and that means stepping away from the old, unhelpful patterns that have kept you STUCK.

Nothing BAD is happening. There's a HUGE difference between THINKING that something BAD is happening and something bad ACTUALLY HAPPENING!

You're just out of BALANCE. Let's get you SORTED.

WORKING DAY I

- FORGIVE yourself for feeling this way. Actually, there's NOTHING to forgive! See it that way. YOU HAVEN'T DONE ANYTHING WRONG! YOU ARE NOT BEING PUNISHED!

  I absolutely promise you that nothing BAD is happening! Yes, the sensations may be unsettling but there is no actual DANGER. It's just the way you're INTERPRETING the sensations that causes you to feel anxious. What if you didn't FEAR it?

- It's important that you give yourself HOPE and OPTIMISM now. Look FORWARD to feeling better. Get EXCITED about that!

- Acknowledge that you arrived at ANXIETY via a lot of NEGATIVITY, WORRY and PESSIMISM. Acknowledge this but DO NOT BEAT YOURSELF UP ABOUT IT!

- Go EASY on yourself today! Be COMPASSIONATE. Say: 'I simply didn't KNOW how to handle this. Soon I will — isn't that GREAT?'

- Really PICTURE getting better. Visualise yourself on HOLIDAY or at an OUTING or SOCIAL OCCASION and see yourself ENJOYING it.

- Find an image that generates a FEELING of RELIEF, OPTIMISM or PEACE. Place it where you can see it and say 'THAT's my default position from here on.'

- Now imagine that you've ARRIVED at this place of contentment. Ask yourself:

  What will I be doing differently?
  What will I have let go of?
  How will my outlook have changed?

  Write down your answers.

- Isolate what it is you're REALLY afraid of. Perhaps deep down you don't think you're GOOD ENOUGH. Something like that is usually at the heart of anxiety, so it's not actually the ANXIETY that needs healing; what needs attention is a CORE BELIEF about yourself that causes you to DOUBT yourself and your WORTH. Write down what you discover.

- See your ANXIETY as an EPISODE, rather than a CONDITION.

YOUR MANTRAS FOR DAY 1

'I am a GOOD person whose thoughts get a little CARRIED AWAY. I am not being PUNISHED.'

'Nothing BAD is happening. I just have a THOUGHT that there is.'

'When I don't add ANXIOUS thoughts, anxiety is just PHYSICAL DISCOMFORT.'

'I am about to learn some new SKILLS that will help me feel BETTER.'

'I am willing to HELP MYSELF feel BETTER.'

DAY 2

We're not trying to get RID of ANYTHING!

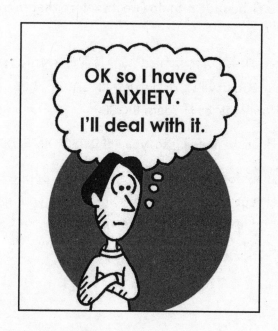

You think you need to ELIMINATE anxiety (also known as 'IT' in my other books) to get BETTER? WRONG! Why? Because you and your anxiety are ONE! If you got rid of your anxiety, you would be carving out a part of YOURSELF!

This is a part of YOU that has become DISTRESSED! Hardly surprising — if someone kept being told the WORST or was CRITICISED endlessly, wouldn't they become DISTRESSED?

That's WHY you feel ANXIETY! IT is telling you you're out of BALANCE. Isn't that HELPFUL information? For now, it's important that you just let it (or 'IT') BE there because IT has a JOB to do (we'll explore that more later).

WISHING IT away, FRETTING over IT, LAMENTING the fact that you have IT, or getting ANGRY or FRUSTRATED with IT only makes IT seem BIGGER!

Why? Because in doing so, you FEED IT. STOP FEEDING IT!

So what to do? Make ROOM for IT. IT has popped up. So be IT. Let IT be there just FOR NOW till you figure IT out and learn what to do. You don't have to LOVE IT or even LIKE IT. Just ACCEPT IT — FOR NOW.

WORKING DAY 2

- IT's here. He's moved in. So be it. Visualise him as an annoying relative who has come to visit for a while. Allocate him a room or his own space and leave him to it.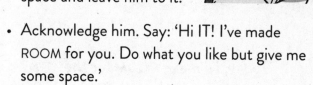

- Acknowledge him. Say: 'Hi IT! I've made ROOM for you. Do what you like but give me some space.'

- Today — DO NOT:

    Read newspapers

    Watch or listen to the news

    Talk about anxiety

    Research anxiety on the Internet

    Read books about anxiety (except THIS ONE!)

- TALK to IT. When IT starts trying to scare you, say 'Yes, thank you for your opinion. Now please go to your room.'

YOUR MANTRAS FOR DAY 2

'Today, I'll make ROOM for the
anxiety to be there.'

'I ACCEPT that this has happened in my life.'

'I'll let IT be as IT IS for the moment
and get on with other things.'

'Today, I won't TALK about IT, OBSESS about IT,
RESEARCH or DISCUSS IT.'

'Today, I'll let IT hang around in
the BACKGROUND.'

DAY 3

It's only
RESISTANCE
to something that
makes it **PAINFUL**

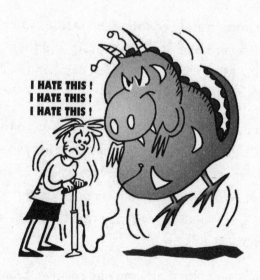

In making ROOM for your anxiety to be as it is and to be in your life at the moment, you have practised the first exercise in NON-RESISTANCE!

Well done! Now let's REFINE that further.

Say you have a really annoying relative who calls or drops in at all hours, prattles on with a whole lot of RUBBISH and generally drives you CRAZY!

Aside from the fact that you haven't set clear BOUNDARIES that she will adhere to (we'll get to that later too!), what can you do?

Practise NON-RESISTANCE!

It works like this. You hear the doorbell and you just KNOW it's her.

You can immediately go into RESISTANCE: 'Oh NO! Not HER again! She'll talk ENDLESSLY and there'll be no getting RID of her!' — in which case, you will end up SUFFERING throughout her visit.

Or, you can take a moment before you go to the door and say 'OK, it's her. I know what she's like, so why would I expect any different? Here we go ...' and open the door. A lot of the STING has gone out of it and — SURPRISE, SURPRISE — you may find that's she's NOT SO ANNOYING this time!

Anxiety is a lot like that annoying relative. Expect it to

be UNSETTLING! Accept that anxiety makes you feel JUMPY. That's how you know you have anxiety!

Besides, it's not the ANXIETY that's causing you GRIEF — it's your RESISTANCE to it.

Another way of seeing how RESISTANCE disempowers you is to imagine a WILD ELEPHANT was coming straight at you. How well would you fare if you tried tackling it HEAD-ON?

The smartest move would be to simply STEP ASIDE and let it BARGE THROUGH, wouldn't it?

It's the same when dealing with anxiety — STEP ASIDE (by not getting caught up in a whole mental drama about it) and let it roll past and wait till it runs out of steam.

In fact, we can take this idea of NON-RESISTANCE even further. Here's a THOUGHT:

RECOVERY is not meant to be HARD WORK! It is not a TEST or a TRIAL but a way to help you feel BETTER! If you think recovery is all about STRUGGLE and SACRIFICE, you're heading in the OPPOSITE direction to feeling BETTER! You're in RESISTANCE!

Feeling BETTER is simply that, and the only other option is to feel WORSE, isn't it? (Or stay STUCK and get nowhere.)

If you see this process as a TASK, it will feel like a TASK. If you see it as a BENEFIT, you will feel better about it, you'll feel more inclined to DO IT and may even come to ENJOY it.

Resistance is PUSHING AGAINST something. If you are PUSHING against, RESENTING or RESISTING it, PUTTING IT OFF or AVOIDING it, you have RESISTANCE going; and there is no PROGRESS to be made when you're in resistance.

Search for a feeling that feels more like RELIEF than EFFORT and you'll be on track.

WORKING DAY 3

- Write down all the things that IRRITATE, UPSET or ANNOY you.

- Do you REALLY need to add them to your stockpile of WORRIES? Are they WORTH it?

- If you find yourself 'EFFORTING', recognise that you're off track, so leave it for a while and do something else.

  The 'something else' might be:

  Reading

  Watching a film

  Taking a walk

  Having a nap

  Having a bath

  Making a warm drink

  Making a meal

  Now return to the task.

  Feel the DIFFERENCE between PUSHING THROUGH and STARTING AFRESH.

- Say 'YES' to EVERYTHING! Say 'Yes, Anxiety — I hear you.'

- If you have a problem that needs a solution and you're feeling OVERWHELMED, walk away and do something else (see above) until you feel you're relaxed enough to FIND a solution. Pushing through is PUSHING through!

- Try doing a normally boring or annoying chore, WITHOUT RESISTANCE (singing along to some great music while doing the dishes works for me!).

- If you're feeling anxious, SING, HUM, WHISTLE or DANCE (yes, it really works!).

- In general: REST MORE, PLAY MORE, PAT YOUR DOG MORE, STROKE YOUR CAT MORE, ENJOY YOUR GARDEN / KIDS / SUNSETS / FULL MOONS / MUSIC / GOOD FOOD / FAVOURITE THINGS MORE.

- AMPLIFY that which SOOTHES; RELEASE that which JARS.

YOUR MANTRAS FOR DAY 3

'I know what anxiety feels like.
No surprises there.'

'When I feel IT, I'll just say
"Oh, YOU again!" '

'My new motto is: "IT IS AS IT IS"
or "SO BE IT"
(and I will shrug my shoulders when I say it!).'

DAY 4

The
magical art
of LIST-MAKING

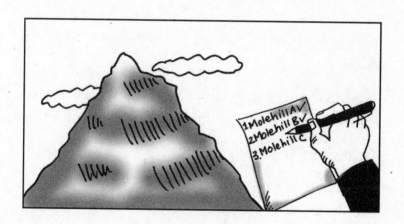

A big contributor to ANXIETY is getting yourself OVERWHELMED!

It's vitally important — especially in the early stages of this work — that you don't GET AHEAD of yourself, or add a whole pile of EXPECTATIONS, PREDICTIONS and DETAILS which will send you into a SPIN.

So, let's keep it SIMPLE.

Don't complicate your RECOVERY process by trying to move mountains overnight — take it ONE BABY STEP AT A TIME. Stop DOING TOO MUCH in your daily life. And give up obsessing about the BIG PICTURE before you've even made sense of the LITTLE PICTURE!

And when you PACE yourself, you have a better chance of staying CALM and actually getting things DONE!

Now, in the early stages of anxiety, or if the anxiety is quite STRONG, you might find it hard to do much at all.

No problem (non-resistance, OK?) — just do WHAT YOU CAN.

ANY problem, no matter how overwhelming it may seem in its ENTIRETY, becomes much more manageable when you BREAK IT DOWN into bits that you can handle. And working through any problem is a PROCESS.

A great (in fact, I find it almost MAGICAL) way to achieve this is via the humble, yet ingeniously powerful, LIST.

Why is that? Because a LIST helps you FOCUS. It helps you sort out what's really IMPORTANT and worth your ENERGY and what you can leave till another time!

AND — when you COMPLETE your list — you realise you were actually capable of doing much MORE than you might have thought.

Here's the truly MAGICAL part: you FORGOT to be ANXIOUS while you were working through the list!

WORKING DAY 4

- Make a list of EVERYTHING you plan to achieve today — and I mean EVERYTHING!

- When you first set out and if your anxiety is HIGH, your list might be as simple as:

    Have shower

    Eat breakfast

    Get dressed

    Clean teeth, etc

    (The order of these items may be interchangeable.)

    Then do a list of what you're going to get done TODAY. Not a *TO DO* list, but a list of what WILL get DONE!

    You might even enter in there the 3 previous days' exercises or some AFFIRMATIONS that you'll spend time on. Or you might allocate some time to focus on something that actually makes you feel GOOD for a change (I highly recommend that you do!).

- List your GOALS. It has been well documented that those who clearly set out their goals are more likely to ACHIEVE them!

Now here's the thing — NOBODY'S GOING ANYWHERE UNTIL THAT LIST IS DONE! You do not move on to the next item until the PREVIOUS item is completed!

Then, at the end of today, I want you to read back over all those TICKED items on your list and give yourself a BIG PAT ON THE BACK!

And while you're at it, notice how your anxiety was a little LESS when you got on with the jobs at hand. What does THAT tell you?

- If you're CONSUMED by worries, make a list of each item you'll worry about. Allocate a WORRY TIME LIMIT of no more than 10 minutes, then be DONE with it!

YOUR MANTRAS FOR DAY 4

'*Gonna do my LIST!*'

'*And I will also do LISTS from HERE ON ...*'

DAY 5

An alien has LANDED

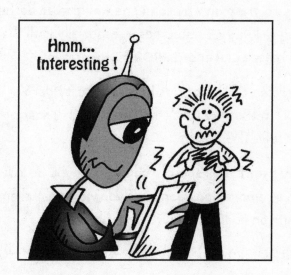

Imagine an ALIEN has just landed on Earth and knows nothing about human EMOTIONS and is curious to explore how humans 'do' emotions.

This alien decides to make you and your ANXIETY a case study and will report back its findings to Alien HQ.

The alien has no concept of ANXIETY. It has absolutely no idea how humans can get so worked up about things or WHY they do in the first place. It's used to just showing up, seeing what happens and responding accordingly.

It has no grasp on why someone would even bother trying to PREDICT outcomes — especially if all that did was create FEAR and TERROR in the present.

To tell the truth, it finds humans pretty darn WEIRD in the way that they seem to LIKE scaring themselves!

Today's work is all about studying how you do YOU from a removed position, as if you were that alien looking on and OBSERVING your behaviour.

Get INTERESTED in yourself, how you FEEL and HOW you come to feel that way.

It is simply not possible to move from one emotional state to the next without an INTERVENING THOUGHT that takes you to the new emotional place.

For instance, I can't suddenly get to feeling ANGRY from feeling NEUTRAL without TELLING myself there's something to be ANGRY about!

It's the same with ANXIETY. There's a thought you're entertaining that says there's something to FEAR or be WORRIED about and so you feel ANXIOUS.

Your THOUGHTS determine how you FEEL. Today, just NOTICE the way it works for you.

NOTICE how you respond to things and, out of interest, notice how the people who seem CALM respond to things. Be CURIOUS. Find out how this works.

Get INTERESTED but DO NOT JUDGE YOURSELF!

You don't have to DO anything about what you're FEELING — just NOTICE and LEARN from it.

Today's work is all about gaining AWARENESS and INSIGHT into your way of responding to stimuli.

You may notice that you have something that is commonly linked to anxiety and is known as a *catastrophic misinterpretation of physical sensations*.

In simpler terms, this means that you tend to see DISASTER in even minor physical changes, such as a change in temperature.

You may notice that there is some CORE BELIEF that you keep returning to when you're anxious, such as 'I'm not GOOD ENOUGH'.

See all that you discover as useful data for your survey of you.

WORKING DAY 5

On the following page is a log to help you do your study of you. Use it regularly throughout the day. (The table at the top is an example of how you might fill it in.) This will tell you a great deal about your THOUGHTS and RESPONSES and their relationship to how anxious you FEEL.

Some things you may discover are:

- That your anxiety FLUCTUATES (i.e. is not CONSTANT).

- That there is a clear relationship between your THOUGHTS and feeling ANXIOUS (even if those thoughts are ABOUT feeling anxious!).

- That you tend to RESPOND in a HABITUAL way to *stressors* (and this can change).

- That your way of RESPONDING is either HELPFUL or UNHELPFUL in alleviating your anxiety.

- That others who find life less stressful have different ways of RESPONDING to stimuli than you, and you can LEARN from this.

INTERESTING, yes?

How I Do Anxiety Study Chart

Example:

Time	Activity	Thoughts	Anxiety (out of 10)	Response
9.15 am	On bus	I'm late!	7/10	Worried more
2.00 pm	At work (Boss angry)	It's my fault!	6/10	Tried to please
6.00 pm	Making dinner	Not thinking	1/10	Carried on

Time	Activity	Thoughts	Anxiety (out of 10)	Response

YOUR MANTRAS FOR DAY 5

'I will step back from myself and notice how I RESPOND to the world.'

'I will notice when I REACT and the things I REACT to.'

'I will notice the THOUGHTS I have when I feel ANXIOUS.'

'I will observe and LEARN from people who are more RELAXED than me.'

DAY 6

Managing the Monkey

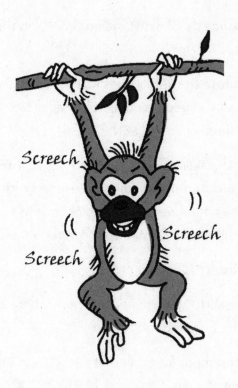

Consider for a moment the INCREDIBLE MACHINE that you walk around in. It's really quite MIRACULOUS how it HEALS from injury, seeks to BALANCE imbalances and ADJUSTS to all kinds of junk that we feed it — including our NEGATIVE THOUGHTS.

Your BODY and BRAIN work extremely hard to keep you in equilibrium and there's a fair bit of leeway in how far you take things, but eventually ENOUGH is ENOUGH; and you have reached that point now!

Did you notice that I didn't include 'MIND' in that statement?

This is because the BRAIN does its best to rebalance, but if the MIND keeps sending it barrages of scary stories, it simply can't RESET!

The more the MIND finds to WORRY about, the more the BRAIN must obediently respond with the appropriate neural responses and chemicals to deal with DANGER — even when that danger is IMAGINED.

The end result? Ongoing ANXIETY!

So, it's the MIND that we need to rein in here and YOU are the one who has to do this.

Tune in for a moment to all that CHATTER in your head. Take notice of what it's saying. Nothing GOOD, eh? You wish it would SHUT UP but on it goes — *screech,*

screech, screech: 'This is BAD', 'That is SCARY', 'It's all HOPELESS', 'Something BAD is going to happen', 'I'm stuck with this FOREVER' and so on.

Sometimes the messages become very PERSONAL and DAMNING: 'I'm an IDIOT', 'I'm a LOSER', 'I'm not GOOD ENOUGH', 'Who would WANT me when I'm like THIS?'

In Eastern philosophy, this is known as 'Monkey Mind'. Here is how Wikipedia describes Monkey Mind:

> **Mind monkey** or **monkey mind**, from Chinese xinyuan and Sino-Japanese shin'en 心猿 [lit. 'heart-/mind-monkey'], is a Buddhist term meaning 'unsettled; restless; capricious; whimsical; fanciful; inconstant; confused; indecisive; uncontrollable'.

There's a story that illustrates the way Monkey Mind works and it goes like this:

There was once a monkey who had been locked in a tower.

When he first arrived, he was hysterical — he raced from wall to wall, scratched at the door, screeched for help and tore out his hair in despair.

Eventually, once he had exhausted himself and calmed down, he started to see the tower differently. He noticed that it was actually quite peaceful. He could look out of the window and enjoy the view of the sky and the trees. He didn't have to answer to anyone nor follow any rules, and for a while he was content — until boredom set in and the walls seemed to close in on him again and he was off in hysterics once more.

There are a couple of points to this story:

1. Your thoughts, and the MOODS that follow them, are never STATIC. What is terrible one day will be pleasant (or bearable) another day and then something else on yet another day.

2. Your OPINION of things is all that governs how they FEEL to you. The tower remained exactly as it was — it was the way the monkey THOUGHT about the tower that changed how it felt to him: one minute a prison; the next a sanctuary. Which opinion was true? Both and neither.

3. Monkey Mind settles down when you give it something BETTER to do.

4. Monkey Mind is loudest when you take NOTICE of it and especially when you BELIEVE what it says!

WORKING DAY 6

- Know that your monkey CAN be (and needs to be) TAMED. If you let him run amok as he has been doing, without any focus or discipline, you can expect more of the same. You need to let him know who's BOSS!

- Open a CONVERSATION with your monkey. After all, he's just a scared little creature! Find out exactly what he's UPSET about.

- How can you SOOTHE his FEARS?
  How might you REASSURE him?
  How might you DISTRACT him?

- TUNE HIM OUT. If you let him BOTHER you, he'll keep going. Treat the chatter as BACKGROUND NOISE — annoying, but not important or even relevant.

  Think about it — does the fact that you're running 10 minutes late for an appointment really mean that you're a HORRIBLE, SELFISH person who can't be TRUSTED with ANYTHING?

  Mostly what Monkey Mind is spouting is NEGATIVE, SUPERSTITIOUS NONSENSE, so why are you taking it SERIOUSLY?

- The best way to quieten your monkey is to quieten YOURSELF, and the fastest and most effective way to do that is through MEDITATION.

You only need 15 minutes' meditation a day to make a HUGE difference to your wellbeing and to significantly quieten your monkey.

Meditation can be as simple as sitting quietly and emptying your mind as much as possible. You can do so by focusing on your BREATH and only your breath. Each time a thought comes, calmly go back to your breath.

Quiet music or chanting 'OM' is also helpful. But if the thoughts are intrusive, a good stand-by is to focus on the words:

NO THOUGHT

Try a 'walking meditation', where you simply go for a walk and focus COMPLETELY on what your feet are doing and nothing else.

Above all, don't WORK at meditation. Just LET GO of Monkey Mind and ENJOY the QUIET.

YOUR MANTRAS FOR DAY 6

'These are just THOUGHTS — not FACTS.'

'I no longer ATTACH to these thoughts.'

DAY 7

Present (un) tense

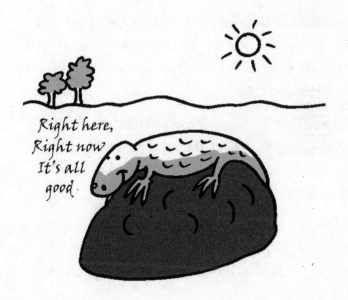

Right here,
Right now
It's all
good.

Here's a statement to reflect on today:

> *You cannot feel anger, resentment or regret in the PRESENT without focusing on the PAST.*

> *You cannot feel fear or anxiety in the PRESENT without projecting into the FUTURE.*

If you're experiencing DEPRESSION, you are spending an awful lot of time in the PAST. When you have ANXIETY, you're spending an awful lot of time predicting the FUTURE.

How about living NOW?

Think about all the DISASTERS you predicted that scared the HELL out of you! How many came TRUE? I hate to tell you but you'd be best not going for a job on a Psychic Line!

What if you let your mind stay RIGHT HERE, RIGHT NOW, doing this thing, then the next thing, moving from one moment to the next, letting each unfold AS THEY WILL.

Worrying ahead of time does nothing except EXHAUST you before you even GET THERE! WORRYING has absolutely no influence on creating a positive OUTCOME!

Staying in the PRESENT is its own form of MEDITATION and it helps on many levels — most importantly, it teaches you to TRUST that things have their own way of WORKING OUT if you just GET OUT OF YOUR OWN WAY!

They also have a better chance of working out if you RELAX and let solutions COME TO YOU.

So let's get into the NOW!

WORKING DAY 7

- Today, be fully CONSCIOUS of EVERYTHING around you.

  Focus on each of the five senses in turn:

  What can you hear?
  What can you smell?
  What can you see?
  What can you taste?
  What can you feel?

- Become FULLY AWARE of all that is ALREADY around you that you simply don't notice because your mind is not fully PRESENT to the PRESENT. Take a moment to APPRECIATE what you now see — there are so many more possibilities than this tight little world of anxiety!

- Approach this day in the following way:

  'What if I let go of EXPECTATIONS?'

  'What if I let things UNFOLD in their own way and FIND OUT what comes next?'

  'What if I don't get hung up on particular OUTCOMES but instead consider that there are

more and better OPTIONS and POSSIBILITIES than I can think of when I'm ANXIOUS?'

'What if I decide that whatever eventuates is the RIGHT outcome for today?'

- Show up for the GIG and see what HAPPENS! Say you were going on a MAGICAL MYSTERY TOUR — would you want to know what the 'mystery' was BEFORE you left?

- Wouldn't that take the FUN out of it? Wouldn't that ruin the whole POINT of the exercise?

- Let your day SURPRISE you! And above all — let it PLEASANTLY surprise you! No projecting future DISASTERS!

- Stay in the PRESENT and TRUST that it will all work out (in 99% of cases, it DOES!).

YOUR MANTRA FOR DAY 7

'Things always WORK OUT in the end.'

DAY 8

'Poor Me' Day

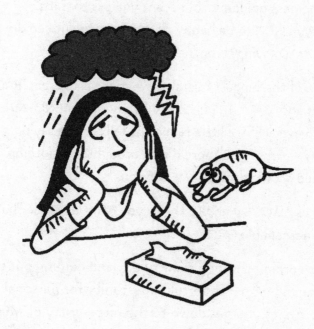

'What's this?' I hear you say. Well, you read it right.

YOU ARE ALLOWED ONE SELF-PITY DAY A MONTH.

There is going to be a day when, no matter how you try, your efforts to lift yourself up fall flat on their faces.

Everything just feels like CRAP and that's all there is to it.

In fact, one of the less helpful aspects of the 'happiness epidemic' of recent years is that it's UNREALISTIC to be happy all the time; and it can drive you MAD trying to be 'up' constantly.

One of the biggest mistakes we make is to treat 'BAD' days and 'CATASTROPHES' as if they were ABNORMAL! 'Into every life, a little rain must fall,' as the saying goes — otherwise there'd be a drought and nothing would grow! It's the SAME for you.

Life is ALWAYS going to throw you CHALLENGES! That's an inescapable FACT.

So, working through a shitty day and coming out the other side is a wonderful opportunity for personal growth, as you get down to the nitty-gritty of what's DRIVING your MISERY (your THINKING and nothing else!) and move on.

See it as having a good old emotional DETOX. After all,

there's no point trying to pour pure water into a contaminated receptacle, is there?

Feeling ANGRY instead? OK, go with that. Get down and DIRTY — but with one NON-NEGOTIABLE condition: YOU DO NOT INFLICT THIS ON ANYONE ELSE, right?

The interesting thing about anger is that no matter how much you try to HIDE it from view, it leaks out ANYWAY, so despite your best efforts to keep a LID on it, innocent bystanders have probably been copping it through a variety of sources — nasty looks, impatient sighs, irritable exchanges or outright tantrums. So you're doing a public service by getting to the heart of this.

The question is: WHO are you angry with? If it's someone else, your anger with them keeps you attached TO them. Do you want to KEEP dragging them around with you?

But almost invariably, it's YOU you're most angry with; in which case, you're going to be unpleasant company to hang out with, so best to flush that out too, by diving deep INTO it!

Not feeling too bad today? GREAT!

Save today's work for another day and move on to Day 9. It's pretty much guaranteed that there will be a day in our month together when you can use these materials.

For those of you ready and primed, GO FOR IT! Don't waste a second of this chance to shamelessly roll around in MISERY or be as much of a CRANKYPANTS as you like — without APOLOGY!

Believe me, it's delightful to give yourself PERMISSION to do so and, when you do, you'll find you sure get SICK OF IT pretty fast!

WORKING DAY 8

- Today's the day to take a 'sickie'. If you really can't do that, then just keep a low profile till you can get some alone time.

  (If that in itself is difficult, you can always add it to the list of things to feel sorry for yourself about!)

  If you have work or other commitments, reschedule your 'Poor Me' day till the weekend.

  Avoid engaging with others any more than is necessary today. Remember that your mood can be CONTAGIOUS and it's your self-pity to do with as you choose without others chipping in with theirs!

- Once you have some ME time, set the stage for a right old PITY PARTY and — here's the thing — you are to INDULGE totally in doing this!

  Get out the following ammunition:

  Journal (if you have one — as in the outpouring kind)

  Old photos

  Old love letters

  Music that makes you sad

Movies that make you sad

Food you shouldn't eat

A MODERATE amount of alcohol (or preferably none — too much makes things a bit too intense and you'll feel WORSE tomorrow)

Tissues, a stuffed toy and a blanket

If you're feeling ANGRY rather than MISERABLE, you'll also need:

A pillow to smash and yell into

Pen and paper to write down all you're ANGRY about. Start with 'I'm angry with X because ...' and let rip!

Or, place a chair opposite you and imagine your 'enemy' (it could be 'IT') sitting facing you and give them a piece of your mind!

- Approach this GUILT-FREE. You are giving yourself PERMISSION to feel crap, instead of thinking you SHOULDN'T feel this way!

- Write down an exhaustive list of EVERYTHING that's WRONG in your world. Do not leave out ANYTHING!

- GRIEVE, RANT, WAIL— whatever! Go for it! The more TEARS the better! Tears are a healthy and natural way to RELEASE.

- Keep going till you're DONE. Ideally, you'll feel TIRED, PURGED and totally OVER feeling SORRY FOR YOURSELF!

  Remember: EVERYONE feels this way at times, but YOU get to RELEASE it in a HEALTHY way!

- Copy the way CHILDREN release their emotions — FURIOUS with you one minute, then climbing onto your lap the next. Once it's OUT, it's DONE!

YOUR MANTRAS FOR DAY 8

'It's not FAIR!'

'Why ME?'

'I'm MAD as HELL and I'm not gonna TAKE it anymore!'

DAY 9

Absolutely
ABSOLUTE-FREE

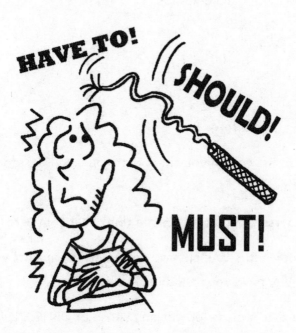

If you've done Day 8 properly, you will probably have gained some breathing space from your emotional CLEAN-OUT.

Excellent — because now we need to really get working on that rotten old 'STINKY THINKING' that has got you deep in doo-doo in the first place!

A great place to start is by eradicating the ABSOLUTES. You can easily live without them! In fact, life will seem a LOT easier when you completely drop these terrorists from your thoughts and speech.

Here are the main culprits:

> *Should*
>
> *Must*
>
> *Have to*
>
> *Ought to*

Think of how often you think that you 'HAVE TO' do something.

Ask yourself: 'What makes me think that I HAVE to?'

Who or what is MAKING you do something against your will? Why have you AGREED to this?

If you take a close look at any sense of OBLIGATION that is running (and ruining) your life, you'll usually find that it's actually YOU who is cracking the whip most of the time!

Does your best friend really CARE if there aren't hospital corners on the sheets when they visit for a cuppa?

Granted, in life there are things that we are required to do to be effective in the physical world, such as being a good employee if we want to keep our job or a good parent if we want our children to feel valued and secure.

Even so, it is the way you MENTALLY approach tasks that causes them to FEEL like a BURDEN instead of a MEANS TO AN END.

I have NEWS for you: you don't HAVE to do ANYTHING! You're not a CHILD; you have FREE WILL, and free will means that you are free to do or not do something!

Freeing yourself from ABSOLUTES in your thoughts and speech is the first step to realising that you actually do have CHOICE and that you can exercise that CHOICE.

You will also come to see how RIGID, LIMITING and DEMANDING living by ABSOLUTES can be.

While we're at it, let's ELIMINATE a few more:

> *Always*
> *Never*
> *No-one*
> *Totally*
> *Absolutely*

See how there's no FLEXIBILITY in these statements? They're ALL or NOTHING, BLACK and WHITE, and also involve a lot of MIND-READING, ASSUMING or GUESSING.

How do you KNOW that NOBODY has EVER done that thing? Have you done a survey?

The simple truth is: you DON'T know. You can only know how it is for YOU.

WORKING DAY 9

- Ask yourself: 'WHY do I think I "HAVE TO"? WHO is cracking the whip?' And if you DON'T do this thing that you feel you 'have to', WHAT THEN?

  You can CHOOSE to — or not to. No-one can really FORCE you. And even if you feel that you are OBLIGATED, how have you ALLOWED that to happen?

  Really get it. Aside from legal and ethical issues, you don't HAVE TO do ANYTHING in this life. Most of the 'obligations' that you feel trapped by are restrictions you have imposed on YOURSELF.

  Practise saying NO. Even if you feel you can't say no to something because the pressure of not doing it would feel too great, then know that you have AGREED to it, and therefore do it WILLINGLY and without resistance.

- AIM to get to a point where you actually feel a little CRINGE if you accidentally use ABSOLUTES or when you observe others using them. You can happily live without ABSOLUTES.

- Try these SUBSTITUTES:

  Could

  Might

  Perhaps

  Want to / don't want to

  Would like to

  Prefer to / not to

  Have decided to / not to

  Would rather not

  It seems to me that

  Occasionally

- Practise finding SOFTER ways of expressing that which would normally constitute an ABSOLUTE.

YOUR
MANTRA
FOR
DAY 9

'Today, I choose to think FLEXIBLY.'

DAY 10

Watch your
LANGUAGE

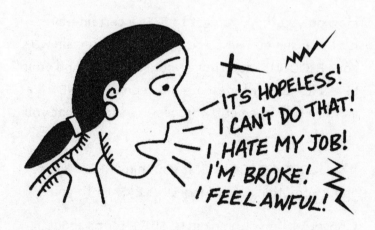

Now that you've had a practice run by mastering ABSOLUTES, today you need to commence what needs to be a LIFETIME COMMITMENT — to be extra careful about EVERY THOUGHT you THINK and EVERY WORD you SAY.

WHY? Because these are the very things that will either keep you ANXIOUS or bring you PEACE. Good reason, eh?

Look at the above statement. Can you see how IMPORTANT it is that, from here on, you choose your THOUGHTS and WORDS carefully? Your words are actually SHAPING YOUR WORLD.

How do you think you get to FEEL a certain way? It's because you THINK about things in a certain way. Your THOUGHTS determine your FEELINGS. And your BRAIN doesn't differentiate between what's REAL or IMAGINED. It obediently processes exactly what you TELL it!

It's not ROCKET SCIENCE! If you think NEGATIVELY about something, it will feel UNPLEASANT to you!

Conversely, if you think in POSITIVE terms about something (or someone!), you look for the GOOD in the situation and you FEEL GOOD about it.

So it's not the THING or the PERSON that causes you to feel GOOD or BAD — it's the way you're THINKING about it or them!

EVERYTHING that we experience in this world is first filtered through our THOUGHTS and BELIEFS.

Whatever you are observing is just AS IT IS (which is neither GOOD nor BAD) until you REPORT it to yourself in a certain way. Then it AFFECTS you in accordance with what you THINK of it — which, after all, is just YOUR opinion!

Whatever OPINION you hold about something is going to determine how you FEEL about it. Nothing EXTERNAL needs to change for you to feel BETTER about something, as you'll see from the exercises.

If you think something's RIGHT, you'll see it as RIGHT. If you think it's WRONG, you'll see it that way. The thing itself has nothing to do with it. It's just being a THING.

We put labels on pretty much EVERYTHING in our world.

This is NICE, that's NASTY, that's BAD, this is GOOD and so on, and these opinions are generated by:

> *Conditioning*
> *Upbringing*
> *Past experiences*
> *Certain expectations*
> *Personal preferences*

We hold on to these beliefs as if we are the sole arbiters of the TRUTH. When you have a BELIEF, you look for EVIDENCE to PROVE IT and you'll reject anything that doesn't fit that BELIEF. And a BELIEF is just a THOUGHT that you've told yourself enough times to make it seem as though it is a FACT. It's NOT. It's still just a BELIEF, which is an OPINION you've THOUGHT and/or EXPRESSED.

You might say, 'But I'm just telling it like it is.' But does acknowledging those so-called 'facts' help you FEEL BETTER?

Being a 'realist' is HELPFUL if it leads you to actively seek a SOLUTION. OBSESSING about a problem or something you can't FIX is just SELF-TORTURE.

'Watching your language' leads to SEEING evidence that the way you think and speak actually influences what SHOWS UP in your experience!

WORKING DAY 10

YOUR AIM TODAY IS SIMPLY TO HELP YOURSELF FEEL BETTER BY THINKING BETTER!

- Sit somewhere where you can observe other people discreetly for at least 15 minutes.

  Look at the first person you see and tell yourself, 'I don't LIKE that person.' Notice how that person appears to you now, once you've decided you don't like him/her. Notice any IMPERFECTIONS that strike you.

  Now do the REVERSE. Tell yourself you like that person. Notice what you appreciate or accept about that person, now that you have decided to like him/her.

  The PERSON hasn't changed. The only change was your OPINION of that person.

  AND ... you have done this with EVERYTHING you have formed an OPINION of in your life!

- Write down your current OPINIONS about ANXIETY. Do they EASE the anxiety or make it WORSE?

Now write down some other possible ways to see anxiety as though you were:

> *A friend who is easygoing*
> *A person who has had anxiety*
> *but has recovered*

- Watch out for any thoughts or conversations that are:

> *Self-deprecating*
> *Judgmental*
> *Negative*
> *Pessimistic*
> *Complaining about anxiety*
> *(in particular, how 'BAD' it is)*

- Practise SUBSTITUTING the above with statements that are:

> *Uplifting*
> *Positive*
> *Optimistic*
> *Helpful*
> *Soothing*

- If you find yourself tempted to report something NEGATIVELY to yourself or others, consider whether you are actually being 'REALISTIC' or 'PESSIMISTIC'.

- Explore the POWER of your imagination. The next time you are about to eat a piece of CAKE, imagine that a FLY has crawled all over it. Do you still want to eat it? Why not? There was no FLY! This is how your THOUGHTS influence your EXPERIENCE. Handle them with CARE!

- Learn APPRECIATION. Take a fresh look at ordinary items around you — your CAR, TV or the HOUSE you live in. Now consider this: someone DESIGNED this. Someone BUILT this. Someone had a JOB because of this. Someone DREAMT of this. Notice how it SERVES you or brings you MOBILITY, ENTERTAINMENT or REFUGE. Appreciate these gifts.

- At the end of today, write down everything GOOD that happened.

YOUR MANTRA FOR DAY 10

*'I choose to entertain
only thoughts that help me
feel UPLIFTED.'*

DAY 11

BELIEVE it or NOT!

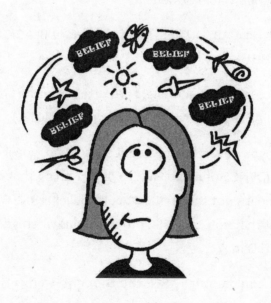

Imagine if your thoughts actually took on PHYSICAL FORM. Some would be BEAUTIFUL; others would be NASTY!

Now imagine that BELIEFS are thoughts that you INVEST in and REPEAT enough to the point where they become ROCK-HARD objects that are particularly stubborn to shift.

You may have INHERITED some of your beliefs through family and therefore these ideas may go back through entire GENERATIONS without ever having been questioned.

Beliefs (like ABSOLUTES) tend to be very BLACK and WHITE.

As discussed earlier, beliefs are often misinterpreted as being FACTS. They're not — they're OPINIONS.

And if you have a BELIEF about something, you'll look for EVIDENCE of it and FILTER OUT anything that doesn't fit it. So it's not that any particular belief is RIGHT — it's just that you can't SEE other options when you are INVESTED in it.

If you could actually SEE the thought-things that you create with ANXIETY, they would look like the entire collection of space junk generated since space travel began!

Wouldn't it be a good idea to take stock of what you decide to UNLEASH into your orbit from here on?

If your THOUGHTS and BELIEFS are PESSIMISTIC, NEGATIVE, ANGRY, ANXIOUS, etc, you'll find your reality MATCHES these concepts.

Examples of BELIEFS about ANXIETY are:

> *Anxiety is bad*
>
> *I shouldn't have anxiety*
>
> *Having anxiety means there is something wrong with me*
>
> *Strong, successful people don't get anxiety*
>
> *I can never get over this anxiety*
>
> *I must have done something wrong to have this anxiety*
>
> *I am being punished by anxiety*

Can you identify with many of the items on this list?

Do you see that the biggest issue is that you have treated these BELIEFS as FACTS?

Sometimes you have company who invest in the same beliefs. Observe any group of family members, co-workers or friends and you will see SHARED BELIEFS tossed around like confetti.

In fact, you're most likely to hang out with people who SHARE similar beliefs to you. All well and good if you're pouring energy into HELPFUL beliefs, but not so good if the beliefs are LIMITING, JUDGMENTAL or DAMAGING.

The beauty of BELIEFS is that when you change THEM you change your EXPERIENCE! For example, if you change a belief that you are UNLUCKY to a belief that says you are FORTUNATE, you'll look for and find evidence that you are fortunate.

Whatever you tell yourself is TRUE will be what shows up, simply because it ALIGNS with your EXPECTATIONS.

Can you see the POWER of this if you use it WISELY?

Change your BELIEFS and you change your WORLD!

WORKING DAY 11

- List some of your BELIEFS about the following:

    Anxiety

    My future

    My past

    Love

    Recovery

    Life

- Reflect on the above in terms of how these BELIEFS have affected your EXPERIENCE.

- Today, OBSERVE the beliefs (disguised as FACTS) that people express so often in their daily lives. Ask yourself: 'Are these FACTS or OPINIONS?'

- If you catch yourself embracing a NEGATIVE BELIEF, simply ask yourself: 'Is this HELPFUL?'

- Try adopting a new belief and look for EVIDENCE to support it. For example: 'People are KIND to me in many ways.'

- Picture your most STUBBORN, NEGATIVE BELIEFS as solid blobs or monsters. Now ZAP them!

YOUR MANTRAS FOR DAY 11

'Today, I choose to *BELIEVE that ALL IS WELL.*'

'Today, I choose to *BELIEVE that I am OK.*'

DAY 12

So,
WHAT IF?

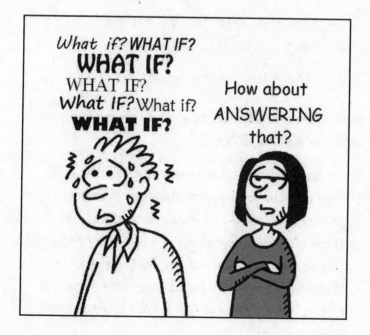

Surely THE mantra for anxiety is 'What if?'

> *What if I fail?*
> *What if I make a fool of myself?*
> *What if they don't like me?*
> *What if he leaves me?*
> *What if it all goes wrong?*

The 'What ifs' can become even more extreme at times:

> *What if I have (insert terrible terminal illness)?*
> *What if my entire family is wiped out?*
> *What if I spend the rest of my life alone?*
> *What if this bridge falls down?*

You can be running late for a job interview and suddenly it's World War III!

I'm late! What if I can't make it at all? What if they give the job to someone else? What if I go broke? What if I have to live on the streets? What if I lose everything — I'll be smelly and ugly and no-one will want me and what if there's a World War — there'll be no-one to help me and I'll be all alone and everything will be gone and I won't survive!

OK, HOLD EVERYTHING!

Remember all we've explored about the way that you 'report' things to yourself?

This is NOT exactly going to EASE your anxiety, is it?

And, as we've also explored, your REALITY tends to match up with your THOUGHTS and BELIEFS.

I'm not saying that you can invoke a plane crash or World War III just by thinking about it (that takes a long, concerted and hugely collaborative effort!), but you CAN bring MORE trouble into your arena because TROUBLE is what you're FOCUSING on (or at least your focus on trouble has DISTRACTED you from being efficient!).

So, you're sitting behind a row of cars that is lined up at a level crossing and the signals seem to be stuck and then, after an eternity, when guys in orange vests have finally got the boom-gates working again, you're in such a STATE that you accelerate too fast and hit the guy in front of you, and because you've been so sleep-deprived, worrying about this job interview, you realise you've forgotten to renew your insurance, the battery is flat on your phone and you just want to curl up into a ball and cry.

Okay, so let's back up a little — let's start again at the 'What if?'

What if you approached things DIFFERENTLY from the start?

What if, instead of the BE-ALL AND END-ALL, you saw the interview as ONE possibility in a world of INFINITE possibilities and if you're MEANT for this job, then you'll get it! If not, you will have done your BEST (and no-one can ask for MORE than your best) and a BETTER option is waiting for you.

Take an EXTREME example of a 'What if?' — a plane crash.

What if you're on a crashing plane? Well, you'll do what you'll do on a crashing plane, which is — since you are NOT currently on a crashing plane — completely UNPREDICTABLE! So why even bother GOING THERE?

WORKING DAY 12

- Write down all the WHAT IFs you have been TORTURING yourself with.

- The best antidote to the WHAT IF? question is to ANSWER IT! OK, so WHAT IF the 'WORST' actually happens? (It SELDOM does, by the way!) Write down 'the worst that can happen'.

  Now answer these questions:

  > *How would you handle the 'worst'?*
  > *What actions would you take?*
  > *Would it really be the end of everything?*

- Today, EXPECT things to TURN OUT IN YOUR FAVOUR, TRUST THEY WILL and SIT BACK and watch how things UNFOLD and SOLUTIONS present themselves.

- Today, if you find yourself worrying, ask yourself: 'Does worrying about this HELP? Does it make one IOTA of difference?'

- WHAT IF it's not really such a BIG DEAL after all?

- Have you actually turned FIVE MINUTES of trouble into a WHOLE DAY of disaster?

YOUR MANTRA FOR DAY 12

'Today, I'll just show up and SEE WHAT HAPPENS.'

DAY 13

Talk IT up

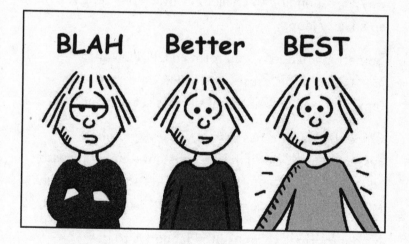

By seeking (and finding) a CALMER way of dealing with the WHAT IF? scenarios, you are learning to RESPOND rather than REACT to *stressors* which would normally send you off the EDGE.

Well done!

Let's keep up that momentum today.

First up, we need to take a look at what we're aiming to ACHIEVE through moderating your responses.

Until now, you have had a HABITUAL (read 'kneejerk') way of responding to challenges which has kept you in an anxiety loop.

Something happens, you form an OPINION that it's 'BAD' and this causes you to FEEL a certain way (anxious), and your internal alarm is set on 'DANGER'.

Once the 'danger' has passed, ideally, the whole system RESETS. But if you're constantly tinkering with NEGATIVE THOUGHTS, WORRIES or RELIVING unpleasant MEMORIES, the system can stay STUCK on RED ALERT.

If your 'normal' response to 'danger' is to get ANXIOUS, over time that becomes the 'normal' place to go, so it takes LESS and LESS to send you there!

So today's work is to take yourself to a DIFFERENT mental place if you feel STRESSED.

If you can change your RESPONSE to one that DISSOLVES the negativity and SOOTHES or GROUNDS you, and you learn to do this more OFTEN, you will be REPROGRAMMING your brain to take you to a more PEACEFUL reaction more quickly.

In time, if you do this OFTEN and CONSISTENTLY, you will build a mental BRIDGE to the better-feeling place and the old bridge to anxiety will fall away.

No matter what's going on, it's important to realise that you can't even SEE a SOLUTION if you're knee-deep in the PROBLEM! You'll get to the solution when you're CALM enough to stand apart from it and RECOGNISE it!

If you are finding it difficult to land on something UPLIFTING, find small things to APPRECIATE such as a colour that you like, or by recalling a good book or movie. Go as GENERAL as you can in your thinking — thoughts that feel STABLE and SETTLING and keep resetting your mind to that equilibrium. With practice that will become your go-to place!

WORKING DAY 13

- If a PROBLEM presents itself, remind yourself that it's a HASSLE, not a DISASTER!

- If you're knee-deep in a PROBLEM, walk away. LEAVE IT till you're RECEPTIVE to a SOLUTION. Meanwhile —

  Take a walk

  Have a nap

  Distract yourself

  Do something else

- Working through any problem is simply a PROCESS. Use the below exercise to help you move closer to where you WANT to be.

  Instead of COMPLAINING (internally or externally) about how HARD something feels to you, TALK IT UP! Say 'Watch how I TURN THIS AROUND!' Then look for ways to DO that!

  Move towards your goal by writing down thoughts that help you FEEL your way towards the End Point.

My job
stresses me

Perhaps I
could set a
deadline to stay or go

In the meantime,
I'll look around

I do like the security
my job gives me, though

And I like SOME
aspects of my job;
I could focus on those

I ENJOY my work

- Here is a great and simple technique loosely based on the natural therapy technique called Kinesiology.

  Call up a MODERATELY troublesome thought that you'd be better off without.

  Cup it in your hands. Now rub your hands together (keeping good contact between the hands) while saying:

  This idea (or memory) can't hurt me. It's the MEANING I give it that hurts me. It has TAUGHT me something. I am WISER because of it. Now its job is DONE. I am here RIGHT NOW watching it dissolve into NOTHINGNESS in my hands in this MOMENT. I am now FREE of this. It's no longer important enough to even think about.

Now, to lock that down, without moving your head, look to the RIGHT, then LEFT, then look DOWN. Done! It's as EASY as that! You can do this as things ARISE and they can be cleaned off before they STICK!

YOUR MANTRAS FOR DAY 13

'I approach challenges calmly and work through them ONE STEP at a TIME.'

'There is ALWAYS a way through.'

DAY 14

Draw
IT
out

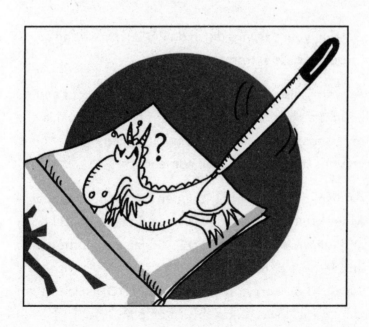

OK, relax — you don't have to be REMBRANDT!

Years ago, I was going through one of those BIG life changes, which involved a lot of heavy emotions and sleepless nights.

At the time, my friend was studying ART THERAPY and I asked her about what she was learning.

The two main things that struck me were:

DRAW LIKE A CHILD DOES — not for the RESULT, but for the EXPRESSION.

And, most IMPORTANTLY — be willing to make a MESS!

Getting your feelings down on PAPER, by writing or through art, is extremely HEALING.

After my discussion with my friend, I raced out and bought a sketchbook and EVERY medium I could lay my hands on — paints, pencils, blow-pens, glitter pens, crayons, felt markers, you name it.

And so, night after night, when I couldn't sleep, or when I felt overwhelmed, I turned to my sketchbook and let WHATEVER WANTED TO COME OUT come out, and — here's the most IMPORTANT thing — without JUDGING or worrying about what ANYONE ELSE might think of it. I was doing this to help ME.

After a while, I actually became EXCITED by what surprises might emerge each night. And I also found that while some of the images were dark or heavy, there were other times when something beautiful, tender or soft came through.

Out flowed 96 pages in two weeks and at the end of this time, something had changed. I felt BETTER, LIGHTER and CALMER.

Now it's your turn. No-one is going to JUDGE what you produce; no-one is going to see it except you. So, go for it. Make a beautiful MESS! You can always start another PAGE!

WORKING DAY 14

- Set yourself up with some art materials. You don't need to break the bank to do this — there are plenty of items you can find in the stationery aisle at your supermarket or in your child's bedroom or schoolbag.

- Get EXCITED by this. You are about to make some discoveries, as well as LET GO of some internal junk you don't need anymore.

- Begin by choosing COLOURS that express how you're feeling and simply start putting them down on paper. Just let the colours go where they want to. Now add anything you like.

- Try drawing your 'IT'. See him/her/it for what he/she/it is — just a little CHARACTER on the page.

- You might like to draw DREAMS or PAST EXPERIENCES you would like to EXORCISE by pouring them onto the page.

- You might like to add WORDS, or write a little about your thoughts on these experiences.

- Draw yourself feeling HAPPY and at PEACE.

YOUR
MANTRA
FOR
DAY 14

'It feels GOOD to let this OUT.'

DAY 15

Rescue me

NOTE: You'll need an hour of quiet,
undisturbed time for today's work.

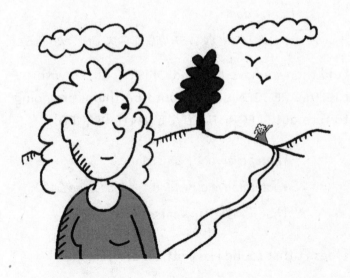

Regardless of your current AGE, when you're ANXIOUS, it's actually a LITTLE KID inside you who is feeling it!

Think about it. Do your REALLY feel like a GROWN-UP when you're ANXIOUS, WORRIED, OVERWHELMED or in DESPAIR?

Reflect for a moment on the NATURE of anxious thinking. Let's be HONEST — isn't it a little 'childish'?

For example, take thoughts such as:

> 'They're all BETTER than me!'
>
> 'I'm USELESS!'
>
> 'What if they don't LIKE me?'
>
> 'I'm NEVER going to get better!'
>
> 'I CAN'T do it!'
>
> 'I'm BAD / WRONG / STUPID / UGLY / UNLOVEABLE etc.'

And then we have the TERRORISING of self with NIGHTMARE SCENARIOS about how things are going to turn out BEFORE THEY'VE EVEN HAPPENED!

> 'What if everybody LEAVES me?'
>
> 'What if I have a HORRIBLE disease and DIE?'
>
> 'What if NOBODY wants me?'

Doesn't that sound like a little kid? Well it IS!

Inside everyone is an Inner Child. Yours is just running wild and that's because there is no GROWN-UP helping them to cope with life!

No WONDER they're scared!

Sometime ago they became stuck in the idea that they were less than PERFECT — probably because someone TOLD them that they weren't GOOD enough and they came to BELIEVE it!

This caused the child to feel UNWORTHY, INSECURE and ... ANXIOUS. And, because these feelings were so INTENSE, a part of you remained STUCK back there!

The ANXIOUS part of you is still that frightened little kid trying to cope in a grown-up's body!

You need to go back and RESCUE the child and help them feel SAFE.

The child needs to know that you will TAKE CARE of them from here on and give to this part of yourself all that you looked to OTHERS to provide.

Be OPEN to letting your FEELINGS come to the surface. This is a TURNING POINT for many people.

WORKING DAY 15

- WITHOUT JUDGING YOURSELF, recognise that you're in CHILD MODE — especially when you're ANXIOUS.

- Also recognise that your Inner Child cannot feel SAFE unless the 'ADULT you' looks after them.

- Get out a photo of yourself as a child and STUDY it. (If you don't have a photo, simply picture yourself as a young child.) Look at the little person that you were. See how you were:

  Innocent

  Open

  Trusting

  Playful

  Hopeful

  Vulnerable

  Small

  ... and DESERVING of all good things

- Picture your Inner Child standing before you right now.

  Is the child well-cared for or scruffy?

What is the attitude of the child towards you?

Is the child happy?

Now tell the child this:

'I've come back for you. I'm sorry I left you behind. I'm going to look after you so you feel safe from here on.'

- Let your emotions around this surface. GRIEVE if you feel inclined to. Release all the HURT, SADNESS and UNEXPRESSED ANGER that has been trapped back then.

- With your NON-DOMINANT hand (i.e. the hand you DON'T normally write with), have LITTLE YOU write you a letter saying how they feel.

YOUR
MANTRA
FOR
DAY 15

'I welcome back the CHILD in ME.'

(For tomorrow's work, you'll need to get a plain-paper book with a nice cover which is specially reserved for this work. You can easily pick up books like this at bargain stores. Find one that looks a little 'special' to you.)

DAY 16

Welcome
HOME!

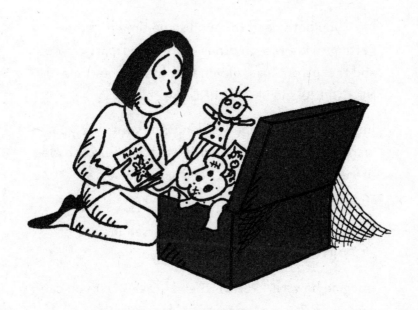

Meeting your Inner Child can bring up many EMOTIONS.

You may have had a little (or even a big) CRY when you saw him/her.

You may have felt SAD or even a little GUILTY that you had left them UNSUPPORTED. Or you may have even felt a bit DISTANT to the child — as if you didn't really KNOW them. In turn, the child may have felt ABANDONED by you and may have expressed that.

All of the above (and any other variation) is perfectly NORMAL. It simply reflects the relationship you have with this vulnerable part of YOURSELF.

Now you both need to spend some time together getting to know each other — the 'child' part of you and the 'parent' part of you that has the new role of NURTURING and PROTECTING the child.

Imagine if you stopped making everyone else your 'parents' or 'authority figures' (that's where the idea of 'have to' comes from!) and saw yourself as EQUAL to others.

Imagine really LOOKING AFTER yourself instead of HOPING that others will do it FOR you!

Imagine how INDEPENDENT and CONFIDENT you can feel when you are 'stepping up' for yourself.

THAT's what this work is about. That's how you can start to make POWERFUL changes in your life. This is VERY IMPORTANT in helping you feel less anxious.

You can also learn to set clearer BOUNDARIES around what you are willing to take on board from here on.

If you are coming from a place that says, 'Nobody gets to treat my kid like that!', imagine how little NONSENSE you'll put up with from now on!

When you have a more CONNECTED and LOVING relationship with yourself, you'll expect the BEST for you and your little kid and you'll settle for nothing less than KINDNESS and RESPECT.

And that goes for your THOUGHTS, too!

Why on Earth would you TORTURE that vulnerable part of yourself with HORROR STORIES?

OK, time to hang out with LITTLE YOU!

WORKING DAY 16

- First and foremost, you need to STOP SCARING THE CHILD! You also need to STOP BULLYING THE CHILD!

- Now get out that photo of you when you were little and put it in a PROMINENT PLACE where you will see it often during the day.

- Your aim is to help the child feel WELCOME, SAFE and INCLUDED in your life, so the more ATTENTION you give to them, the better will be the BOND with YOURSELF.

- Using your lovely new 'special' book, create a 'Welcome Home' book for LITTLE YOU. In this you might draw or write down the things that were special to you as a child. You might even like to cut out pictures from magazines and paste them there.

  Your book might contain:

  Photos of childhood
  Drawings or pictures of favourite toys
  Special keepsakes and mementos

Memories of favourite:

- *People*
- *Activities*
- *Places*
- *Clothes*
- *Foods*
- *Flowers*
- *Games*
- *Movies*
- *Books*
- *TV shows*
- *Music*

- Decorate it as you wish, but remember: the more effort you put into making this CONNECTION, the better you will FEEL!

- Talk to LITTLE YOU. ASK for THEIR opinion. INCLUDE them as much as possible in your everyday life.

YOUR
MANTRAS
FOR
DAY 16

'When I am at PEACE with myself,
I am at PEACE with all.'

'When I am my own CHAMPION,
I don't need others to be.'

DAY 17

'I've got your BACK!'

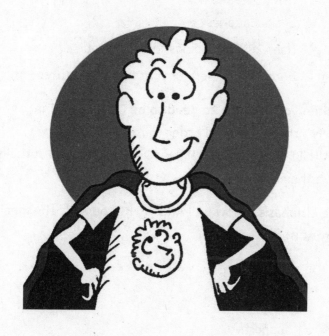

When there has been a FRACTURE between you and your Inner Child and the child has felt ABANDONED or left to deal with all the responsibilities of life by him/ herself, it's going to take a while for them to TRUST you to STEP UP in their best interests.

Up to this point, if you haven't:

> *Spoken up for yourself*
> *Looked after yourself*
> *Taken responsibility for your choices*
> *Worked through problems without flipping out*
> *Kept on top of your chores and responsibilities*
> *Set boundaries*
> *Been kind or compassionate to yourself*
> *Forgiven yourself for your human mistakes*

... then you're going to need to be CONSISTENT in DOING these things in order to restore TRUST in YOURSELF and to help LITTLE YOU feel that you actually have their BACK!

The emphasis is now on PARENTING yourself. The ideal parent is:

> *Understanding*
> *Caring*
> *Supportive*

Creates a sense of stability
Gets things done
Sets healthy limits
... and looks after you!

There is a set of NEEDS that, if attended to, will help you and LITTLE YOU feel secure in the world. They are:

Love

Security

Boundaries

Attention

Rest

Play

Approval

Hope

No-one else can cater to these needs for you as well as YOU can because YOU KNOW BEST how you FEEL, what you LIKE or DISLIKE and what SATISIFIES you.

No-one else SHOULD do this for you (yes, I've used the 's' word! — it's a rarity!) because it's simply NOT THEIR JOB!

Others can COMPLIMENT you, of course, and you them, but it's you who is living in YOUR body and living YOUR life.

You may find that you have strengths in catering to some of the needs on the list but weaknesses in others, or you may need to do some serious catching-up on ALL of them!

That's OK — remember, it's a PROCESS.

When you become your own CHAMPION, SUPPORTER and BEST FRIEND, you NEED less from others. When you give to yourself that which you may never have been given, you are HEALING an old wound, without relying on others to change in order for it to heal.

LITTLE YOU has a role to play, too. Let them restore your sense of WONDER, CURIOSITY and PLAYFULNESS.

This is CRUCIAL WORK so, please, GIVE IT YOUR ALL!

WORKING DAY 17

- Today (and do this EVERY DAY from here on),
  begin by making an AGREEMENT with LITTLE YOU.

  The agreement covers the PRACTICALITIES
  that need to be attended to in daily life by the
  ADULT and some ENJOYMENT and RELAXATION
  for the CHILD.

  Your AGREEMENT may go something like this:

  'I'm going to work so that we have MONEY,
  somewhere to LIVE and FOOD to eat, but I'll be
  home by 6 p.m. and then we'll take a walk and
  later we'll watch our favourite show till bedtime.'

  Then BE home by 6 p.m. Go for a walk (because
  you said you would) and make sure you enjoy
  some relaxation and rest time. Add in a little
  TREAT to really keep the child happy!

  You need to STICK TO THE AGREEMENT! That's
  how LITTLE YOU comes to TRUST you.

- Work through the following list of NEEDS,
  noting how each applies to you and your
  approach to life. ATTENDING to these needs as
  you would for your own child, helps YOU feel
  SAFE and SECURE:

NEEDS	EXAMPLE RESPONSES
LOVE	*Am I as kind and nurturing to myself as I would be to a real-life child? Do I love myself?*
SECURITY	*Do I have enough material security to feel safe? Am I on top of that?*
BOUNDARIES	*Do I say NO enough? Do I protect myself by setting limits?*
ATTENTION	*Do I look after myself well? Do I attend to my physical needs (hunger, rest, thirst, etc) promptly?*
REST	*Do I give myself time out when I need it?*
PLAY	*How can I fit more fun into my life?*
APPROVAL	*Do I give myself enough pats on the back?*
HOPE	*What can I look forward to and get excited about?*

- Today, take time to view the world through a CHILD'S EYES. MARVEL at the world around you — the clouds in the sky, the dog walking with its owner, the sound of wind in the leaves. Look for the wonder in ordinary things. It's EVERYWHERE!

- If you feel ANXIOUS, know that it's just LITTLE YOU reminding you that you're out of BALANCE because you're:

    Overdoing things
    Judging yourself
    Thinking negatively
    Not looking after LITTLE YOU!

YOUR
MANTRA
FOR
DAY 17

*'Hey Little Me,
I'm HERE FOR YOU!'*

(You might want to do a little planning and preparation for tomorrow's process, which is PAMPER DAY! Read through 'Working Day 18' for ideas.)

DAY 18

Pamper
Day!

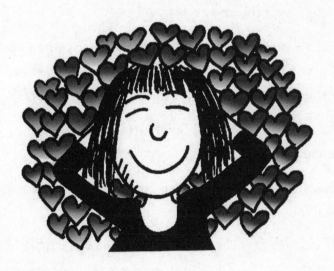

After all this DEEP STUFF, it's time for you (and LITTLE YOU) to have a lovely day of INDULGENCE!

You may want to schedule this for a day off so that you can really go the whole hog; but even if you're WORKING, it is possible to do this in a way that allows you to enjoy some little LUXURIES and down-time.

There is MORE to this than might appear on the surface. By putting yourself FIRST (for once!), you are acknowledging your WORTH and you are giving your Inner Child the much-awaited ATTENTION that they have yearned for all this time.

And why is this so IMPORTANT?

Well, you've EXPERIENCED what happens when your Inner Child is NEGLECTED, haven't you? Or when others' needs or your 'duties' are your priority?

You become ANXIOUS! Surely THAT'S motivation enough!

Because if you DON'T attend to your Inner Child, they will soon become a BRAT!

If you're not giving yourself enough ATTENTION, APPRECIATION, APPROVAL or AFFECTION, your LITTLE YOU will make things extremely uncomfortable until you're FORCED into taking care of yourself!

Your Inner Child can make you:

Sick

Burnt out

Prone to tantrums

Depressed

and ... Anxious!

So be NICE to yourself. Today is a day to really FEEL how GOOD that can feel.

Use your IMAGINATION to come up with some beautiful ways to show your APPRECIATION to yourself for being the AMAZING person you really are!

Today is YOUR day.

Enjoy! (And your LITTLE KID will be DELIGHTED, too!)

WORKING DAY 18

- Enjoy a sleep-in if you have the day off.

- Spend some time just appreciating the MORNING — the light, the sounds, nature.

- Start the day with a HEALTHY breakfast. Make it from the BEST ingredients.

- If you're working, LEAVE your desk at lunchtime! Dine-in at a café or take your lunch to a park.

- If you have the day off, schedule some TREATS. Some suggestions are:

    Massage or facial

    Manicure or pedicure

    Movies

    Window shopping

    Road trip

    Visit a gallery/museum

    Go to an ice-cream parlour

    Bushwalk

    Swim

    Read a novel

    Play a musical instrument

Whatever you FANCY!

YOUR
MANTRA
FOR
DAY 18

'I'm WORTH it!'

DAY 19

Say 'Thank You'!

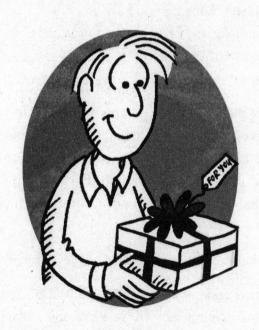

Religion has promoted it for CENTURIES and now science has endorsed it: people who feel and express GRATITUDE are generally more CONTENT and have a greater sense of WELLBEING than those who don't.

Gratitude releases FEEL-GOOD HORMONES such as *dopamine*, *serotonin* and *oxytocin* and helps build deeper personal connections.

But here's the thing — being grateful REALLY works, even when you can't see any reason to be!

Although you may feel like the UNLUCKIEST person on the planet because you have anxiety, if you want to see some quick-fire improvements, it's time to get some GRATITUDE!

'What do I have to be GRATEFUL for?' you ask. 'My dog died, I lost my job, my boyfriend left me, I'm broke ...' and so you list all the things that are WRONG in your life and THEY become your entire focus. It then SEEMS as though there is nothing GOOD happening, let alone things for which you might be GRATEFUL.

Well, what DO you have to be GRATEFUL for?

Well, for a start, you are HOLDING THIS BOOK in your hands (or reading it on some electronic device) which means that (a) you had enough MONEY to BUY it; (b) someone CARED for you enough to GIVE it to you; or (c) you have access to a library that TRUSTS you enough to lend you its books or use its computers!

And I imagine that if you're able to buy or download this book, you have a ROOF over your head, FOOD in your belly, CLOTHES to wear, a SOURCE OF INCOME and the FREE TIME to read it — all of which is more than many people on the planet have.

When you start looking for things to be GRATEFUL for (or at least to APPRECIATE), you'll find that there are actually many things of value in your life that you have simply taken for GRANTED.

The FASTEST way to feel BETTER about almost EVERYTHING is to be GRATEFUL for it and, believe it or not, that includes ANXIETY!

'Whaat?!!'

If you hadn't experienced ANXIETY, would you be making the changes you're making now for the BETTER? Would you be in a place where you are FORCED to address that which has not been working for you?

Would you know how to recognise that you're out of BALANCE and how to FIX that?

GRATITUDE helps you to:

> Stop focusing on the NEGATIVE
>
> Find the BEST in a tough situation
> (thereby easing it and creating solutions)
>
> AMP UP your good-feeling chemicals
>
> Be more GENEROUS
>
> Get out of YOURSELF
>
> APPRECIATE things

And the beauty of this is — the more you GIVE it, the more you GET it back!

WORKING DAY 19

- Being GRATEFUL is a CHOICE. CHOOSE to be grateful today.

- Do something nice for others as often as possible today. Examples are:

  Write to someone expressing your appreciation

  Thank service people you encounter

  Compliment someone

  Give way to a driver

- Post an expression of APPRECIATION for something on Facebook (e.g. 'Beautiful sunrise today').

- BAN all whingeing or complaining today!

- Start a GRATITUDE JOURNAL. Begin by listing:

  Three things to thank yourself for doing well today

  Three things that went well today

  Three things in your life that you are grateful for

  Three people who have been kind to you or have supported you

And take it from there. See how many more things you can ADD to the list each day.

- THANK your ANXIETY! Say 'Hey, thanks for LOOKING OUT for me!' (because ALL your IT is doing is trying to keep you SAFE!).

- Recall a DIFFICULT time from the past. Obviously you got through it. Be GRATEFUL for the way you OVERCAME this. You can do it AGAIN!

- AMPLIFY your APPRECIATION of GOOD things, such as the TASTE of food, the SMELL of NATURE, the LOVE that your friends, family, partner and/or pet offer(s) you.

YOUR
MANTRA
FOR
DAY 19

'Thank you!'

DAY 20

Laugh
IT
off

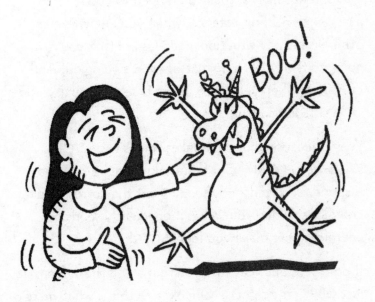

Good grief, you do take life terribly SERIOUSLY, don't you? What if you DIDN'T?

Today, you're going to LIGHTEN UP. In fact, the best skill I can teach you is to learn to be CASUAL about anxiety, because you've got into this fix by being so very EARNEST about everything!

All those memes about a noble fight against ANXIETY are just DRAMATISING it. It's not going to be such a BIG DEAL if you stop MAKING IT a big deal!

First up, let's take a look at an interesting aspect of finding the funny side, even in DIRE circumstances.

Your EXPRESSION actually dictates how you FEEL to a large extent! For instance, when you FROWN in an otherwise happy situation, chances are that you're going to feel DOWN, no matter what's going on! And of course, when you SMILE in the face of adversity, the OPPOSITE is also true.

Why? Because your brain takes things very LITERALLY! When you FROWN, your brain thinks you're SAD and responds accordingly by sending out the corresponding chemicals. When you SMILE, it obediently sends out chemicals that make you feel BETTER!

It doesn't QUESTION why you're making these faces, it just OBEYS the signals. 'Oh, okay — this is what we're feeling now.'

LAUGHTER THERAPY has gained enormous popularity in recent years and you may even consider joining a group.

The BOTTOM LINE is that the body and mind LOVE laughter! Laughter releases more of those FEEL-GOOD CHEMICALS — such as *endorphins* — so it's worth a shot.

Even if you can't get a full belly laugh going today, try SMILING more.

Your IMAGINATION is a STRENGTH. Use it to VISUALISE feeling GOOD, and your BODY and MIND will follow.

And here's the beauty of this: you can't be LAUGHING and ANXIOUS at the SAME TIME!

If you're able to have a bit of a laugh at your anxious self, *GOP The Guru of Panic* — my cartoon creation on Instagram — is a wry look at just how we can get ourselves in a tizz. #guruofpanicqa

WORKING DAY 20

- Tell someone a JOKE today. Here are a few jokes to get you started:

  'Anxiety is a great cardio workout!'

  'Not sure if it's anxiety or whether the sky is actually about to fall.'

  'Thanks for the invitation, but let me overthink about it and let you know.'

  'Thought I might stay anxious till something comes along to be anxious about.'

  'What are you anxious about?' 'Everything!' 'At least you're democratic.'

  'Hey, guess what? I've learned how to be calm and anxious at the same time!'

- Have a gentle laugh AT YOURSELF and how 'out there' your anxious thoughts can get.

- Close your eyes and go inside and recall (or imagine) a time when you felt really ALIVE, at PEACE and were absolutely CONTENT with yourself, others and the world. This particular memory has been reserved for EXACTLY this moment and this purpose. FEEL it fully in your body. AMPLIFY that feeling. BASK in the glow of it. From here on, you can call on this memory ANYTIME you LIKE.

- Now think of a time when you were laughing so HARD that tears were pouring down your cheeks. Your belly hurt from laughing, your cheeks were aching. Feel it bubbling up inside till you actually find yourself laughing in the same way. You can also use this ANYTIME you need to!

- Put on your favourite FUNNY movie. Remember: it's simply not POSSIBLE to be feeling GOOD and feeling ANXIOUS at the same time!

YOUR
MANTRA
FOR
DAY 20

*'I refuse to take
ANYTHING seriously today.'*

(To prepare for Day 21, you might like to read the next
chapter through in advance.)

DAY 21

You're
SWEET
enough

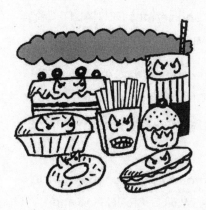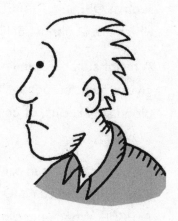

People drastically underestimate how much the type of FOOD they consume impacts on their EMOTIONS!

It's extraordinary that we dismiss the connection between the FUEL that we put into our bodies and how WELL our body functions (including our EMOTIONAL state).

If you put rubbish fuel in your car, would you be surprised if it BROKE DOWN? Of course not! In fact, you'd see it as INEVITABLE.

By far the biggest culprit in our modern diet is SUGAR.

High sugar consumption has proven to be the major cause of a range of diseases (many PREVENTABLE), such as OBESITY, DIABETES and serious DENTAL DECAY, which are at almost EPIDEMIC proportions globally.

A hit of sugar — similar to other ADDICTIVE DRUGS — gives you a temporary 'HIGH', creating a spike in your blood sugar. But, of course, what goes UP must come DOWN!

A SUGAR CRASH can cause you to experience symptoms such as IRRITABILITY, MOOD SWINGS, BRAIN FOG and FATIGUE. When your blood sugar dips, you may find yourself feeling ANXIOUS or DEPRESSED.

Sugar-rich and carb-laden foods can also mess with the *neurotransmitters* that help keep our moods stable.

Consuming sugar stimulates the release of the mood-boosting neurotransmitter *serotonin*.

Constantly over-activating these serotonin pathways, however, can deplete our limited supplies of serotonin; this can also contribute to symptoms of depression.

Sugar isn't restricted to just the obvious SWEETS, DESSERTS and CAKES; it is also in any highly processed, starchy food, such as PASTA, WHITE RICE and WHITE FLOUR.

Just out of interest, take a stroll around your supermarket and you'll see how manufacturers keep you hooked by adding sugar to just about EVERYTHING — even SAVOURY dishes!

It would be a good idea to do some research on this subject, but for today we're just going to do a little 'tidy-up': avoid or, at the very least, severely limit SUGAR, CAFFEINE, ALCOHOL and JUNK today!

Good grief, people — you can do it for ONE DAY! Think of it this way: you're not 'SACRIFICING' anything; you're doing something NICE for your poor, exhausted, overwhelmed system. It needs a REST. Give it one!

WORKING DAY 21

- The instructions for today are SIMPLE: be MINDFUL of what you're putting into your BODY!

- Eat good, HEALTHY, NUTRITIOUS FOOD today — wholegrains, fresh vegetables, a small amount of fresh fruit (don't overdo the fruit — it also contains sugar) and a light serving of meat (if you must — going without meat today would be ideal as meat is harder for the body to digest).

- Drink plenty of WATER (avoid pre-packaged juices and soft drinks).

- Do a bit of RESEARCH on the effects of sugar on mood and consider adjusting your LIFESTYLE accordingly.

- Note how you feel at the end of today.

YOUR MANTRA FOR DAY 21

'I'm LOOKING AFTER myself.'

DAY 22

The two-letter word

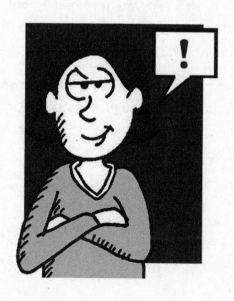

Now you've learned how to look after YOU and LITTLE YOU better, we move on to a major ANXIETY-PROVOKING area of dealing with OTHERS.

Chances are, if you've had a hard time because you feel that people have:

> *Ripped you off*
> *Taken you for granted*
> *Been rude to you*
> *Bullied you*
> *Taken liberties*
> *Ignored your needs*

... then it's most likely you have really wobbly BOUNDARIES, and the one word you need to exercise more is the little power-packed missile 'NO'.

If people are walking all over you, it's because you haven't said it OFTEN enough, LOUDLY enough, CLEARLY enough or with enough CONVICTION to be heard and taken SERIOUSLY.

'But,' you say, 'I say NO all the time but no-one listens!'

You may say the word but it may not have the right amount of POWER in it. Too much force and you'll get people's BACKS UP. Not enough 'oomph' and nothing will change.

An effective 'NO' doesn't just involve saying the WORD; it needs to come from the right PLACE, at the right TIME, with the right INTENTION.

The perils of NOT saying NO because you don't want to UPSET anyone are enormous.

If you're saying 'Yes' when you don't really want to, people still think you mean 'Yes'.

You then find yourself stuck in a situation you don't want to be in, seething with resentment because you think that person 'made' you do this thing you hate.

They didn't. You said 'Yes'.

This is PASSIVE AGGRESSION — one of the most DISEMPOWERING of human behaviours.

With passive aggression, you're all SMILES and AGREEABLE at first — you comply, obey, go along with — because you don't want to get anyone OFFSIDE ('See what a good person I am?').

Inevitably though, sooner or later, you feel used and put upon. You SHUT DOWN or become MOODY and ANGRY at those who have 'put you through this', and you resort to little 'sabotages', such as being late or forgetful, as a means of getting your point across.

But others can't figure out what's going on. You were once so FRIENDLY and now you're just acting WEIRD!

They don't understand or completely miss your 'HINTS', which exasperates you even more!

Then, one day, you can't take it anymore and you EXPLODE!

And it's all because you didn't say one little word.

It's time to start saying 'NO'.

WORKING DAY 22

- You do not need anyone else's PERMISSION or AGREEMENT to make your own CHOICES. You do not need to EXPLAIN. You are allowed to have LIMITS. You are allowed to have PERSONAL PREFERENCES.

- Close your eyes and check into yourself and locate a spot somewhere along your sternum that feels GOOD. That spot is YOU. Now FEEL your BOUNDARIES. Feel how far you extend to each SIDE, FRONT and BACK. Feel how ROBUST (or not) your 'area' feels. If it feels 'collapsed', visualise it EXPANDING and GAINING POWER.

- Stand in front of a mirror. Take a deep breath and feel your 'HARA', which is your 'warrior strength', your 'centre', and is situated in your solar plexus. Visualise your hara becoming EMPOWERED and FEARLESS.

- Now quietly but firmly say 'NO'. Study yourself for any tics or give-away signs that tell you that you are not fully centred, such as a frown, raised eyebrows, head turned to the side or even a smile.

- Practise till you feel that your 'NO' comes from quiet strength that gets the message across with CONVICTION and that you MEAN IT.

- This is especially effective if you do it with a friend who can act as your 'coach' and give you feedback as to whether your 'NO' has hit the spot with them or not.

- Keep in mind that saying 'NO' doesn't mean you don't LIKE or LOVE someone. It simply means you have different PREFERENCES.

As one of my wonderful teachers once said: 'You can say ANYTHING if there is LOVE behind it.'

Having love for YOURSELF means you SPEAK UP.

YOUR MANTRA FOR DAY 22

'I can say NO and still LOVE you.'

DAY 23

None of your
BEESWAX

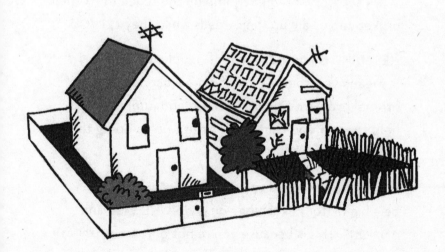

'PEOPLE-PLEASING' is very common in people experiencing anxiety (especially if LITTLE YOU is seeing others as having POWER over you). The main factor in this is a lack of healthy PERSONAL BOUNDARIES.

Personal boundaries are like fences around a house. They define individual 'properties' — in other words, they show the limits of someone's PRIVACY but also the extent of their RESPONSIBILITY.

If you're trying to keep everybody happy (usually at your OWN expense) then you're either letting people wander all over your space, doing whatever they like in YOUR territory, or you're jumping the fence to fix their broken tap or dig up their weeds while they LET YOU.

RESCUING is another form of people-pleasing. It means you spend a lot of time worrying about others' problems, advising them and jumping in to help them if you think they aren't up to doing things themselves.

While this all sounds very NOBLE it can, in fact, be a big factor in keeping you OVERWHELMED and ANXIOUS. This is because you're not only trying to meet your own needs (if at all), but you are also second-guessing the needs of OTHERS.

Freeing yourself from wobbly boundaries is the understanding that you can't really SAVE anyone; nor is it your job. It is also the understanding that what others do is not yours to TAKE ON BOARD, nor CONTROL.

We don't 'GET' people to do things. They either do them or they don't and for their own reasons. No matter how hard you try to CHANGE them, people will do what they think is going to work for THEM.

The only way for a person to solve his or her problem is first to OWN it and take RESPONSIBILTY for it. Not everyone WILL do that but basically, if it's not YOUR problem, it's not yours to SOLVE.

And — think about it — if I'm taking over your problems, then I'm actually saying, 'I know better than you what is best for YOU.' I don't.

Maybe you want someone to change their behaviour because it OFFENDS you. They WON'T. GIVE IT UP.

The only thing you have CONTROL over is how you RESPOND to their behaviour.

When you spend less time worrying about what someone ELSE is doing, you have more time to get YOU sorted!

WORKING DAY 23

- Ask yourself: 'What if I discovered that I absolutely could not RESCUE anyone?' What if it wasn't MY job to fix them but THEIRS?

- Also ask yourself: 'What if I didn't FEAR someone's DISAPPROVAL? Would I be so ACCOMMODATING? What if I saw myself as an EQUAL? SO WHAT if they're annoyed at me?'

- Now pose the question: 'What if speaking MY TRUTH was more IMPORTANT than how it was RECEIVED?'

- Draw a sketch of you as a house with your own 'yard'. Now list the things that are within your LIMITS.

- Tune in to yourself for any feelings of RESENTMENT during an interaction. This is an indication that a boundary has been CROSSED or that you have not set a clear LIMIT.

- If you decide to set some limits today, be CLEAR about what you WANT. No HINTING. Spell it out.

YOUR
MANTRAS
FOR
DAY 23

'I cannot SAVE, FIX or RESCUE
anyone except myself.'

'Today, I will respect people's right to
learn (or not learn) from their MISTAKES,
just as I have that right.'

'I have a RIGHT to ask for
what I WANT.'

DAY 24

You am I

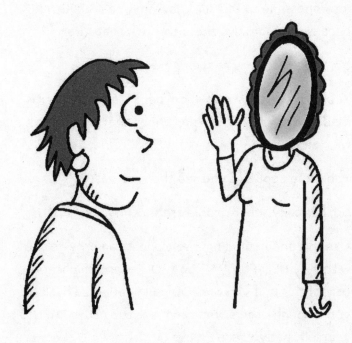

Want to know how well you're TRAVELLING?

Then take a look at the CHARACTERS who wander onto your playing field today.

They're actually showing you YOU!

So, how does this WORK?

Remember that we looked at how we perceive life through our own FILTER of BIASES, PAST EXPERIENCES, CONDITIONING and EXPECTATIONS?

So, if we take that into account, we can see that it's impossible to REALLY know anyone AS THEY ARE because we perceive them through that filter.

So, in a sense, you're seeing YOURSELF!

You're seeing them as 'nice' because your filter is made up of previous experiences that told you this was 'nice'.

The same applies if you see them as 'nasty'.

So, basically, what people are showing you is YOU!

Use this understanding wisely and it can provide you with very HELPFUL INFORMATION — and the beautiful part of this is, if you see YOURSELF reflected back to you through others, you can make the ADJUSTMENTS to yourself that you can't make on them. AND the more ALLOWING, LOVING, FORGIVING and GENEROUS you are to others, the more you are being those things to yourself. It's a WIN-WIN!

You do not need anyone's PERMISSION or APPROVAL to live your life as you CHOOSE. And VICE VERSA. Of course, for every CHOICE there are corresponding CONSEQUENCES, and you're probably very aware of those when you have made an unhelpful choice.

Whether those consequences cause you to feel BETTER or WORSE, they are still the result of the choice YOU made in the first place. It is not something that was DONE to you, even though it might feel that way.

This is a crucial part of recovery. It's called OWNING it. We've all made some UNHELPFUL choices and it's easy to blame OTHERS or CIRCUMSTANCES when it all goes pear-shaped. However, it was YOU who made the choice to respond in a way that SERVED you or not.

Accepting RESPONSIBILITY for where you find yourself instead of blaming others is LIBERATING — because, with this awareness, YOU get to steer your own life from here on and you are not SUBJECT to what others do.

WORKING DAY 24

- Today, as you observe others, take note of how you FEEL about, and interact with, them. What does this tell you about YOU? Especially notice the things you are CRITICAL of in others. Do you do these things yourself? Perhaps you are feeling a little ENVIOUS?

  Examples of seeing yourself in others:

  Are people FRIENDLY to you? If so, in which ways do you INVITE friendliness?
  If people are DISMISSIVE of you, how are you not making yourself VISIBLE?

- Now that you have learned about the Inner Child, see if you can identify the Inner Child in OTHERS. How might this make you feel more COMPASSIONATE towards others (and yourself)? Does this knowledge help you feel more at EASE?

- Also with regard to the Inner Child, notice when you are making others into your PARENTS or AUTHORITY FIGURES. What if you didn't do that anymore?

YOUR MANTRA FOR DAY 24

'I will learn about MYSELF by what others are REFLECTING back to me.'

DAY 25

Nothing COMPARES to YOU

I AM
Gloriously, Magnificently,
Uniquely, Unapologetically

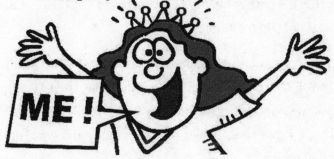

When you don't feel too GREAT about yourself, you'll tend to see others as being SMARTER, WISER, BETTER or more TOGETHER than you.

I have NEWS for you. They're NOT!

You have NO IDEA what someone is really feeling inside and I can pretty much guarantee that there are very few people on this planet who aren't making similar (unfavourable) comparisons about themselves.

Even the wonderful, urbane, intelligent and worldly Clive James revealed in a recent interview that he often felt that 'in a room full of people, I always feel like everyone else is a grown-up but me'.

People with low self-esteem will tend to swing between extremes when comparing themselves to others — either seeing themselves as LACKING in some way or SUPERIOR in others.

When you can see others as your EQUALS, you realise that EVERYONE, without exception, has their strengths and weaknesses, JUST LIKE YOU; and EVERYONE has made some spectacular mistakes along the way (unless they're in a coma!) — JUST LIKE YOU.

However, you are not here to live like anyone else! You are here to live YOUR life in your own UNIQUE way.

You are MEANT to do things DIFFERENTLY from others and you are not meant to turn somersaults so that SOMEONE ELSE can have a perfect life!

Likewise, if you expect others to behave in a way that PLEASES you, you are destined to be DISAPPOINTED because they WON'T. And if you're doing that, then your WELLBEING rests entirely on how someone else behaves, which is, at the very least, PRECARIOUS.

You are MEANT to have certain challenges in order to hone your PARTICULAR skills.

You can ONLY be YOURSELF! What ELSE can you be?

Stop APOLOGISING for being who you are. If someone CRITICISES you, what does it say about THEM? If you can OWN your peculiarities, instead of being offended, you can AGREE with your critics and that will be the end of the discussion. 'Yep, I'm usually late, aren't I?'

ENJOY your WEIRDNESS. OWN it! ACCENTUATE it! Make it an ART FORM!

WORKING DAY 25

- Who are you? What makes you UNIQUE? List all the things that set you APART. How can you make these things POSITIVE ATTRIBUTES?

- OWN it. Go down that list and say 'I AM THAT!' And SMILE when you do so.

- List all the POSITIVE and NEGATIVE aspects of the people you know. See how they BALANCE out?

- Notice what you are CRITICAL of in others. How might this REFLECT something about you?

- Now notice the people who LOVE you. What does this say about YOU?

- List YOUR positives and negatives.

- How might you BUILD on the positives and WORK ON the negatives?

YOUR MANTRA FOR DAY 25

'I AM WHO I AM, and that's a GOOD THING.'

DAY 26

Getting
your
DUCKS
in a
ROW

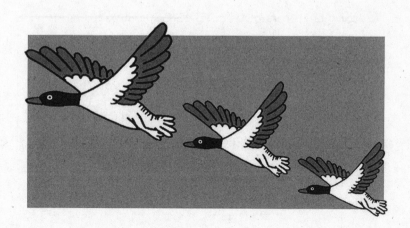

The father of modern psychology, Carl Jung, first coined the term 'synchronicity' which, in simple terms, could be described as 'meaningful coincidences'.

Here are some examples of synchronicity. You finally leave that relationship and the perfect partner appears as if by MAGIC. You've been worried about money for so long, you finally GIVE UP and money suddenly APPEARS. When you think all HOPE is gone, someone happens along who INSPIRES you to keep going.

What is actually happening is not as COINCIDENTAL as it may seem. The things you ASK for do come along, but only when you've LET GO of something that was IN THE WAY!

And the thing that's blocking your way to feeling better is that you keep HANGING ON to ANXIETY!

Getting better involves LETTING GO of anxiety being the PRIORITY, and LINING UP with the things that help you FEEL BETTER. And you have much more INFLUENCE over what comes along than you realise.

Which way are you HEADED with your THOUGHTS? What are you FOCUSED on? Are you pointed TOWARDS anxiety or AWAY from it?

What are you ALIGNED with? Feeling BETTER or feeling WORSE?

RECOVERY isn't going to come to you until you MATCH UP with it!

We're going to explore the basics of ALIGNMENT today.

Here are some concepts to ponder:

1. Your THOUGHTS, and particularly the way they make you FEEL, align you with MORE or LESS of something.

2. You need to be on the same WAVELENGTH as the thing you want to ATTRACT. So if you want to feel BETTER you need to LINE UP with PEACEFUL, SUPPORTIVE, SOOTHING and CALMING people, ideas, activities, thoughts and self-talk.

3. You need to be on the WAVELENGTH of the thing you want, EVEN BEFORE IT ARRIVES! That's how you DRAW it to you. If you feel GOOD about something in advance, it will feel GOOD to you when it ARRIVES!

4. Be clear about what you're saying 'YES' to because THAT'S what you'll line up with. And take note that when you're saying 'NO' to something (e.g. 'I don't want this ANXIETY!'), you're actually saying 'YES' to it, because it has your ATTENTION. So stop making what you DON'T WANT the focus of your attention.

5. There are LIMITLESS POSSIBILITIES, all happening at once, from which you can CHOOSE BEFORE THEY HAPPEN by VISUALISING them. If you have been busy visualising MISERY, STRUGGLE, ANXIETY and PESSIMISM and seeing these as being the only REALITY, then that choice is the equivalent of being at a magnificent banquet and filling your plate only with the food that has gone off and complaining that the banquet was a RIP-OFF!

6. Whatever you're LOOKING FOR, you'll SEE. Whatever you're SEEKING, you'll find.

All day, whether or not you have been AWARE of it, you are ALIGNING with people and experiences that you are a MATCH to. Till now, this has been UNCONSCIOUS. Today is about becoming AWARE of and RESPONSIBLE for what comes your way.

Take a look at what you have attracted so far. Don't like it? Well, you need to get on a DIFFERENT WAVELENGTH — the wavelength of that which you would PREFER to experience.

If you wish to line up with better outcomes, begin by 'reporting' your hopes, dreams and experiences to yourself in a POSITIVE way.

Many people use AFFIRMATIONS for this purpose. Great! But do you realise that you have ALREADY been doing affirmations ALL YOUR LIFE!

Anytime you have thought or said 'This is how something is', you have made an AFFIRMATION. And look what that affirmation MATCHED you with!

Think of how POWERFUL THIS IS! If you successfully apply these principles to achieving RECOVERY, imagine what ELSE you can LINE UP with!

The possibilities are truly LIMITLESS!

WORKING DAY 26

- If you're eating CRUMBS at the BANQUET, choose instead to have only the BEST.

- Think about ways you can ATTRACT more PEACE into your life, starting today.

  For GREATER PEACE OF MIND, for example, you might choose to:

  > Not find fault where you normally would
  > Surrender the need to be 'right' in a discussion
  > Give up on perfectionism

- Have a shot at being the PARKING SPOT KING or QUEEN. EXPECT a spot to show up. DO NOT DOUBT that it will.

- Set your vibe to 'Today is going to be a GOOD DAY' and then look for the ways that it IS a GOOD DAY.

- Pick something small that you would like to ATTRACT. Be SPECIFIC — 'A book about ...' 'A pink scarf', 'Blue earrings'. THINK about it LIGHTLY in a RELAXED and POSITIVE way. The HOW and WHEN of it showing up are not yours to WORRY about. Just TRUST that it will show

up. And it will. Have FUN with this. If you
can attract a RED BUTTON, who says you can't
attract a RED CAR?

YOUR
MANTRA
FOR
DAY 26

'Today, I will open myself up to infinite POSSIBILITIES.'

DAY 27

'Frankly,
my
dear ...'

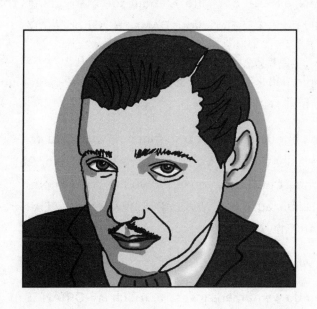

LUCKY YOU! You now have another day off from all this SELF-DISCIPLINE and INNER EXPLORATION!

This is the day when you don't give a DAMN, a HOOT or a [insert expletive here, if that floats your boat]. In other words, you are not to care about anything much at all today!

Dishes not done? Pfft. Hair unwashed? Meh.

However, unlike 'Poor Me' Day, this is not as purely self-indulgent as it might appear at first. This is actually a VERY IMPORTANT day in your progress.

Why? Because, basically, you give way too much of a DAMN, a HOOT or a *#@% about too many things that really don't DESERVE your DAMN, HOOT or *#@%!

You're giving a DAMN, HOOT or *#@% about what people THINK and it needs to stop because it is making you feel ANXIOUS!!!

Think about why you do so much of what you do — especially the stuff you'd really rather NOT do. At the heart of these, you'll find you're doing them either because you WANT APPROVAL or you FEAR DISAPPROVAL.

So, what if you didn't CARE?

Why do we humans invest so much IMPORTANCE in what others think of us?

We haven't evolved much past our ANCIENT ANCESTORS. If the tribe kicked them out, their very SURVIVAL was at risk — from starvation, wild animals and the elements.

Hardly a biggie for us these days with our 24-hour convenience stores, pet shops and central heating.

Of course, we need the company of others to feel whole; but if you're making yourself SICK trying to ensure that everyone else has a PERFECT LIFE, you're OVERDOING it!

So, today you have permission to not give a D, H or *#@%! It's wonderfully LIBERATING — in fact, you may enjoy it so much, you actually make a HABIT of it!

At the very LEAST, you would benefit from being very SELECTIVE about where you invest your D's, H's or *#@%'s from here on.

WORKING DAY 27

- Make a list of ALL the stuff you regularly give a DAMN, HOOT or *#@% about. Leave NOTHING off the list. Be RUTHLESS! This is a total CLEAN-OUT of all those ENERGY-WASTERS.

- Now put a tick next to those things on the list that you do because you give a *#@% what OTHERS might think. These items are FORBIDDEN today.

- Today WEAR whatever you FEEL like wearing. If that's old overalls, pearls or a Halloween wig, so be it. Dare yourself! After all, you don't give a *#@% today, right?

- DUMP all duties except those which are ABSOLUTELY NECESSARY for YOUR wellbeing. YOUR wellbeing, I said!

- Today, do only what you FEEL like doing. Really get in TOUCH with that. (Isn't this FUN?)

- If someone asks you why you haven't done SUCH and SUCH, tell them you don't FEEL like it!

YOUR
MANTRA
FOR
DAY 27

*'Today, I will totally enjoy
not giving a [X].'*

(Substitute X with your choice of word.)

DAY 28

LISTEN
to
YOURSELF!

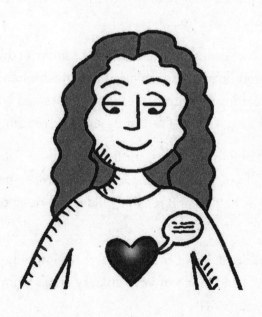

Tune in to that little voice within. No, not THAT one!

The one that speaks calmly and clearly and that you KNOW is the TRUTH (whether you like what you hear or not).

That is the voice of your INTUITION and it needs to be your GUIDE from here on.

It's time to give priority to that 'knowing' over your MIND and its stories — after all, it's all that inner yabber that has tied you up in KNOTS, isn't it?

You've listened to those stories long enough — the stories that say, 'I don't know what to do!' (you do), or 'what if it all goes wrong?' (then you'll have learned something, won't you?).

The MIND causes you to OVERTHINK, and overthinking can tie you up in knots. Think of the times when you've had a clear insight into something then talked yourself out of it as all those FEARS and DOUBTS crept in.

That initial knowing was your INTUITION — or 'gut feeling', if you prefer — and, in order to make better use of this helpful and reliable guide, you need to hone your SKILLS in using it.

As mentioned, like it or not, your intuition tells you the TRUTH and much of your anxiety arises from not LIVING your TRUTH.

Your TRUTH may be that you need to make some changes that you have been putting off (and you KNOW you have), but your RESISTANCE to making those changes is the REAL source of your unrest.

There is no 'bad' message — there's just a message that you'd PREFER to hear or not.

Look, you're constantly making CHOICES anyway, so why not go with the one that feels TRUE, instead of overthinking yourself into a frenzy?

Settle, go within and find out what your INTUITION can tell you.

Be PLAYFUL with this. It can be FUN!

WORKING DAY 28

- Make a list of things you could do today. Now pick the one that you feel DRAWN to. Go with it and see what happens.

- Go on a MAGICAL MYSTERY TOUR! Go for a walk or, better still, if you have a car, go for a drive. Just head off in any direction, with no particular destination in mind. At each intersection, pause, go within and FEEL whether to turn left, right or go straight ahead.

- Keep going till you discover what you were meant to FIND, SEE or HEAR on this outing.

- Bring your ANXIETY into the conversation. It's your guide for what to watch out for. Make USE of your IT instead of fearing IT.

- Say 'Hi IT! Any messages for me today?' Then listen for the answer. IT can ALERT you to when and how you're OUT OF BALANCE.

- LITTLE YOU will also love that you're doing this Let him/her join in, too.

You know how little kids are RUTHLESS truth-tellers? You have one on board. Listen for 'I don't want to hang around with him/her' or

'I don't want to do that; I want to do this.' And check in if that's RIGHT for you.

- Think about moving FORWARD. Ask yourself: 'What would serve me best right now?' Write down what comes to you.

YOUR
MANTRA
FOR
DAY 28

*'I trust that I have the
ANSWERS within me.'*

DAY 29

'End of Story' Day

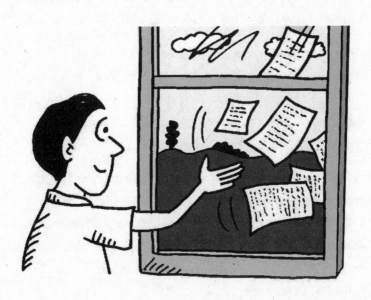

Let's put that old STORY to bed — the one that says 'I'm not GOOD enough' or 'Life is too HARD for me' or 'I'll NEVER get over this.'

Let's clean out the CLOSETS of all the old HEARTBREAK, HEARTACHE and 'this was done to me' stories that keep you from fully stepping into your BEAUTIFUL, POWERFUL, CAPABLE self.

Let's knock on the head all the ideas that ANYTHING ANYONE has done to you (or you to them, for that matter) still holds any POWER over you.

This can only happen if you keep INVESTING in the STORY. You are doing this when you let the past DEFINE you.

How do you see yourself? Be aware of 'I am' statements such as 'I am a VICTIM of ABUSE' and 'I am ANXIOUS', which keep you locked into some past experience. You may have HAD these experiences but WHO YOU ARE is someone beyond that.

When you keep yourself stuck in PAST pain or trouble, recognise that what you're telling yourself is just a STORY about your past. It isn't happening anymore. When you realise the story you're telling is just WORDS and IDEAS, you can throw away the first draft and write a BETTER story from here on.

Besides, that STORY is very biased. GOOD things happened too, but you have filtered them out.

The SAD story or the story of being a VICTIM is very compelling, isn't it? But does it SERVE you anymore?

You've come a long way over these days and we're nearly at the end of our journey together.

Now is the time to leave all that SORROW, TROUBLE, FEAR and HURT behind.

It's DONE. Learn from it and start AFRESH.

It is no longer WHO YOU ARE.

WORKING DAY 29

- Write down the whole MESS. This is the LAST TIME you will let it DEFINE who you are or LIMIT your ability to move forward.

  GRIEVE, RAGE and LET IT GO.

  Now BURN it, SHRED it, BURY it. These are just WORDS on paper. This is just a STORY you've been telling about how you thought it WAS, not how it IS anymore.

- Now write the NEXT chapter of your life story. If you were telling a WHOLE NEW STORY about your PAST, PRESENT and FUTURE, what would you write?

- Today is truly the FIRST DAY OF THE REST OF YOUR LIFE. Make it a celebration. Maybe it's time for a MAKEOVER or a CLEAN-OUT or a DECLUTTER.

- Gather together all these things from the PAST, say goodbye and THROW THEM AWAY.

YOUR
MANTRAS
FOR
DAY 29

'This has been just one CHAPTER in my life story.
It's not the WHOLE BOOK.'

'I now tell a NEW STORY about
MYSELF and my LIFE.'

'I am not what HAPPENED to me.
I am what I choose to BECOME.'

DAY 30

Have a little faith

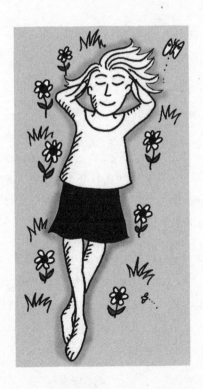

In his wonderful book *Man's Search for Meaning*, Jewish psychiatrist Viktor Frankl describes his time as a prisoner in Auschwitz and the horrors endured by those in the concentration camp.

He observed that those who had a philosophical, religious or spiritual MEANING or CONTEXT for their suffering, such as 'I'm going to live to save others', were more likely to EMOTIONALLY (and PHYSICALLY) survive their ordeal.

If you look for MEANING in your experience with anxiety, the challenges could be seen as:

Necessary motivators

Contrasts

Elements that force change

Lessons

Imbalances to be rebalanced

Having FAITH is often seen as a 'religious' notion, but you can have faith in YOUR LOVED ONES, LIFE ITSELF, THE POWER OF LOVE and so on.

And if you are RELIGIOUS or SPIRITUALLY inclined, your FAITH may have been tested through this time. This is often because of a human tendency to see 'God' or a higher being in HUMAN terms, and whether we see a deity as LOVING or PUNISHING or even ABSENT is often influenced by the AUTHORITY FIGURES in our lives.

If you are one of those people who PRAY, do you EXPECT your prayers to be ANSWERED and look for EVIDENCE that they ARE? THAT'S the magic ingredient. That's FAITH.

Do you have a friend you completely TRUST? Do you lie awake wondering if they'll show up for your lunch date? No. You don't DOUBT it. You KNOW they'll be there. That's FAITH.

Regardless of RELIGION, if you have FAITH that ALL IS WELL — despite all appearances to the contrary — it will be. WHY?

Because when you have FAITH, you can RELAX; you stop trying to CONTROL and let yourself be GUIDED, you're more willing to ACCEPT and LEARN from your experiences and you'll let things unfold as they are DESTINED to.

So, allow yourself a little faith. Have faith in NATURE, knowing that everything ADAPTS and REBALANCES, even after CHAOS. Have FAITH in the basic GOOD in people.

Have faith in your AMAZING, WONDERFUL SELF!

WORKING DAY 30

- Pick a symbol — something you have no RESISTANCE to; for example, it could be a PINK FLOWER, a BLUE BIRD or a YELLOW BICYCLE. Now notice how often this symbol appears today. Find HOPE in this.

- Just for TODAY, try living to the idea of 'Let go and let God' (or FATE or THE UNIVERSE) and feel what a RELIEF it is that YOU don't have to have all the ANSWERS. Leave it to be sorted out WITHOUT you.

- Consider the following notions:

  What if all that you've experienced through anxiety was MEANT TO BE? How have these experiences pushed you to CHANGE for the BETTER? How have you GROWN as a result? What did you need to LET GO OF and now HAVE in its place?

- Write down what your experiences of anxiety have GIVEN YOU in relation to all these things. How can you USE what you now know for the GREATER GOOD?

- Today, feel WORTHY OF LOVE, and bask in the MIRACLE that is LIFE.

YOUR MANTRA FOR DAY 30

'Today, I surrender to the FLOW of life.'

And, so, our work is done. I now say 'Namaste', which means 'The God in me salutes the God in you.'

May you be at peace.

Also by
Bev Aisbett ...

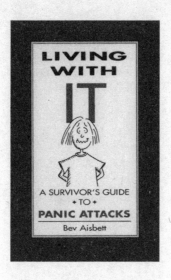

LIVING WITH IT:
A Survivor's Guide to Panic Attacks

Panic attacks — approximately 5% of the population will experience them at sometime or another. Seemingly coming from nowhere, the dread of having an attack itself transforms the ordinary world of everyday life into a nightmare of anxiety and suffering.

In this refreshing and accessible guide, Bev Aisbett, a survivor herself of Panic Syndrome, tells us how panic disorders develop and how to recognise the symptoms. With the aid of her inimitable cartoons, she covers topics such as changing negative thought patterns, seeking professional help and, ultimately, learning skills for recovery. *Living With IT* provides much needed reassurance and support, leading the way out of the maze of panic with humour and the insight of first-hand experience.

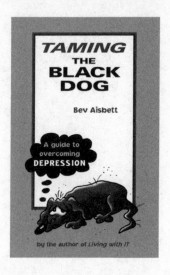

TAMING THE BLACK DOG:
A Guide to Overcoming Depression

Don't want to get out of bed in the morning?

Feeling as though the light is fading at
the end of the tunnel?

You may be suffering from depression, a condition
Winston Churchill referred to as the 'Black Dog'.

Taming the Black Dog is a simple guide to managing
depression, which an estimated 1 in 5 people will
suffer in one form or another at some time in their
lives. Modelled on Bev Aisbett's successful *Living with
IT*, *Taming the Black Dog* has a unique blend of wit
and information, and is an invaluable guide for both
chronic sufferers of depression as well as
anyone with a fit of 'the blues'.

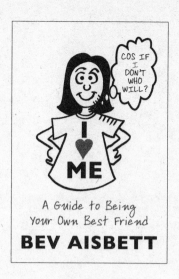

I LOVE ME:
A Guide to Being Your Own Best Friend

Do you feel that life has left you out in the cold?

Do you feel unloved, unwanted or overlooked?

Do you reach out to others for support only to find
that they leave you disappointed or dissatisfied?

There are times in our lives when we seem to have
no-one in our corner, and so we feel depressed, lonely,
hurt or angry. But there is someone to turn to — if
you know how. Someone you can trust and rely on,
no matter what: yourself!

Bev Aisbett, who has helped thousands of Australians
find a way out of depression and anxiety, now shows
you how to find the most loyal friend of all ...YOU!

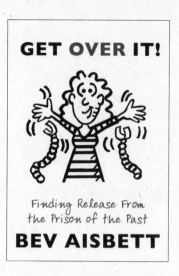

GET OVER IT:
Finding Release from the Prison of the Past

Got difficulties?

Get over it ...

The past can be a prison which traps us in the illusion that life is hard, that we are meant to suffer and that our fate is out of our hands.

'One day I decided that this was an extra burden that I could live without.'

Bev Aisbett once again delivers the straight-talking, compassionate advice that has helped tens of thousands of people move past trauma and into hope.

Get Over IT is the perfect resource to help you feel more grounded in your ability to face the difficulties in your life.

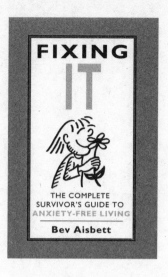

FIXING IT:
The Complete Survivor's Guide to Anxiety-Free Living

What's your IT?

Anger? Fear? Low self-esteem? Depression?
Addiction?

Fixing IT brings together, for the first time in one volume,
a complete guide to surviving anxiety in its many forms
and how to move on to achieve change and growth in our
lives. This single edition includes three titles:

Living with IT: A Survivor's Guide to Panic Attacks
Living IT Up: The Advanced Survivor's
Guide to Anxiety-Free Living
Letting IT Go: Attaining Awareness out of Adversity.